European School of Oncology

Monographs

Series Editor: U. Veronesi

L. Denis (Ed.)

The Medical Management of Prostate Cancer II

With 16 Figures and 23 Tables

Springer-Verlag
Berlin Heidelberg New York
London Paris Tokyo
Hong Kong Barcelona
Budapest

Professor Dr. Louis Denis

Department of Urology
Algemeen Ziekenhuis Middelheim
Lindendreef 1
2020 Antwerp, Belgium

The European School of Oncology gratefully acknowledges sponsorship for the Task Force received from Pharmacia AB, Helsingborg, Sweden, whose engagement in the research on prostate cancer has resulted in the origination and development of estramustine phosphate (Estracyt®) and polyestradiol phosphate (Estradurin®)

ISBN-13: 978-3-642-76280-2 e-ISBN-13: 978-3-642-76278-9
DOI: 10.1007/978-3-642-76278-9

Library of Congress Cataloging-in-Publication Data
The Medical management of prostate cancer II / L. Denis (ed.). p. cm.–(Monographs / European School of Oncology) ISBN 3-540-53443-1 (alk. paper).–ISBN 0-387-53443-1 (alk. paper) 1. Prostate–Cancer. I. Denis, L. II. Title: Medical management of prostate cancer 2. III. Series: Monographs (European School of Oncology) [DNLM: 1. Prostatic Neoplasms–therapy.] RC280.P7M44 1991 616.99'463–dc20 DNLM/DLC

Softcover reprint of the hardcover 1st edition 1991

Bookbinding: J. Schäffer GmbH & Co. KG, Grünstadt
23/3145-543210 – Printed on acid-free paper

Foreword

The European School of Oncology came into existence to respond to a need for information, education and training in the field of the diagnosis and treatment of cancer. There are two main reasons why such an initiative was considered necessary. Firstly, the teaching of oncology requires a rigorously multidisciplinary approach which is difficult for the Universities to put into practice since their system is mainly disciplinary orientated. Secondly, the rate of technological development that impinges on the diagnosis and treatment of cancer has been so rapid that it is not an easy task for medical faculties to adapt their curricula flexibly.

With its residential courses for organ pathologies and the seminars on new techniques (laser, monoclonal antibodies, imaging techniques etc.) or on the principal therapeutic controversies (conservative or mutilating surgery, primary or adjuvant chemotherapy, radiotherapy alone or integrated), it is the ambition of the European School of Oncology to fill a cultural and scientific gap and, thereby, create a bridge between the University and Industry and between these two and daily medical practice.

One of the more recent initiatives of ESO has been the institution of permanent study groups, also called task forces, where a limited number of leading experts are invited to meet once a year with the aim of defining the state of the art and possibly reaching a consensus on future developments in specific fields of oncology.

The ESO Monograph series was designed with the specific purpose of disseminating the results of these study group meetings, and providing concise and updated reviews of the topic discussed.

It was decided to keep the layout relatively simple, in order to restrict the costs and make the monographs available in the shortest possible time, thus overcoming a common problem in medical literature: that of the material being outdated even before publication.

Umberto Veronesi
Chairman Scientific Committee
European School of Oncology

Contents

Introduction

Louis Denis

Department of Urology, Algemeen Ziekenhuis Middelheim, Lindendreef 1, 2020 Antwerp, Belgium

This monograph is composed of a review and edited contributions of a workshop on the Medical Management of Prostate Cancer. The workshop was organised in the framework of the Task Force Programme of the European School of Oncology and supported by an educational grant of Pharmacia Leo Therapeutics AB.

The timing of this second workshop coincided with major advances in our overall insight into the treated natural history of this disease, in new clinical technology for the diagnosis and staging of the disease and in innovative endocrine treatment. In this turmoil of events, one should be aware of the fact that we learned to integrate separate sources of increased knowledge into a clinical approach that will be able to treat the many different forms of prostate cancer according to their prognosis, and, more importantly, to adapt this treatment to each individual patient. Clinical over- and undertreatment is still common and the Task Force feels that each patient is entitled to a tailored treatment where quality of life is weighed against overall treatment. This monograph still deals with advanced prostate cancer, but medical treatment might have to play a role in earlier stages of the disease. The advantage in survival and quality of life of our patients may be real according to the expectations of the expert panel of the European Programme Against Cancer, but major breakthroughs will emerge from actual laboratory research and existing randomised clinical trials. We are not aiming for the magic bullet against cancer, but we are determined to limit the ravages of this disease in our greying male population by closing in on our target of cure or stabilisation of this cancer step by step. It will be a march into the 21st century, but each march has to start with a first step.

It is my privilege, as chairman of the Task Forcce, to thank the faculty for its major and patient effort. It is clear that this work really represents the end result of a broad consensus development in prostate cancer, where many organisations, such as the National Prostate Cancer Project of the U.S.A. - now absorbed into several organisations - and the European Organisation on Research and Treatment of Cancer collaborate with a group of national, active organisations from Japan to Finland. It is appropriate to thank the dozens of experts who contributed in one way or another to our discussions. They are represented by the appropriate references to the manuscripts. In addition, we would like to acknowledge direct scientific support to the preparation of this monograph by Prof. C. La Vecchia of Milan, Prof. O. Maissonneuve of Lyon, Dr. T. Zheng of Lyon, Prof. D.G. Zaridze of Moscow, Dr. S. Zoppi of Milano and Dr. J. Bruynseels of Beerse. The secretarial support of Mrs. R. Denie and, last but not least, the support of the European School of Oncology team, Ms S. McGrath, Ms M. de Jager and Dr. A. Costa, was vital to the completion of the monograph. Ms B. Montenbruck managed to speed the project through the Springer edition with patience and enthusiasm.

The Epidemiology of Prostate Cancer

Peter Boyle

SEARCH Programme, Unit of Analytical Epidemiology, International Agency for Research on Cancer, 150 Cours Albert Thomas, 69372 Lyon Cedex 08, France

Despite it being one of the commonest forms of cancer, relatively little is known about the aetiology of cancer of the prostate. In 1980 it was estimated that prostatic cancer was the fifth most frequent cancer in men, with an estimated 235,800 cases occurring annually worldwide [1]. The incidence continues to increase [2] and incidence and mortality rates of cancer of the prostate demonstrate wide international variation with, for example, a 120-fold difference present between areas of highest and lowest incidence, according to the most recently available statistics [3]. Increases continue to take place in the incidence of prostate cancer in Scotland and Connecticut [4] as well as the Scandinavian countries [5].

The highest incidence rates continue to be observed among blacks in the United States (Table 1): rates in blacks are around 80% higher than rates in whites in the same areas of the United States. Rates in United States whites are the second highest group of rates followed by Scandinavian countries. Within Scandinavia there is considerable variation, with the rates in Sweden more than 50% higher than in Finland [5]. Incidence rates are intermediate in most areas of Europe, being higher in western than in southern and eastern Europe (Fig. 1). The incidence of prostatic cancer is high in Polynesians (native Hawaiians and New Zealand Maori). Prostatic cancer incidence is moderately high in Central and South America and the lowest

Table 1. Cancer incidence rates in blacks and whites in some populations of the United States. Annual, age-adjusted incidence rates per 100,000

	Black	White	Relative risk*		Black	White	Relative risk*
Alameda	100.2	44.5	2.3	Alameda	87.8	49.6	1.8
Bay Area	92.2	47.4	1.9	Bay Area	82.5	50.0	1.7
Los Angeles	79.1	44.3	1.8	Los Angeles	82.6	49.6	1.7
Atlanta	95.7	51.9	1.8	Connecticut	72.3	46.8	1.5
New Orleans	72.1	39.2	1.8	Atlanta	91.2	53.4	1.7
Detroit	73.2	41.4	1.8	New Orleans	71.8	42.0	1.7
				Detroit	91.1	51.2	1.8
(source: Waterhouse et al., 1982 [7])				(source: Muir et al., 1988 [3])			

* blacks relative to whites

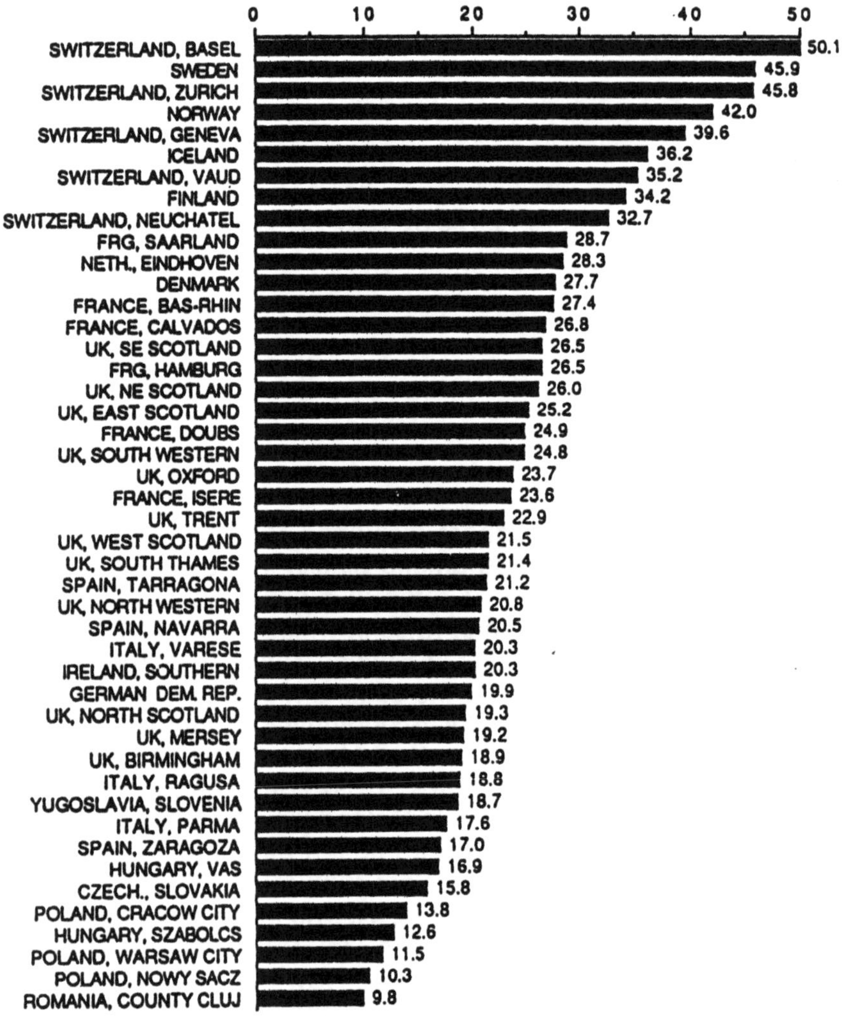

Fig. 1. Incidence of prostate cancer in Europe (average age-standardised incidence rates per 100,000, 1978-82)

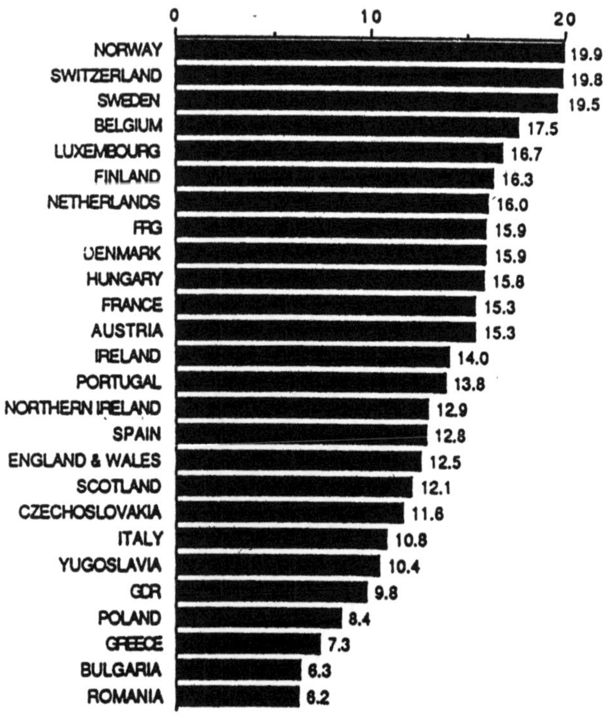

Fig. 2. Mortality from prostate cancer in Europe (average age-standardised mortality rates per 100,000, 1978-82)

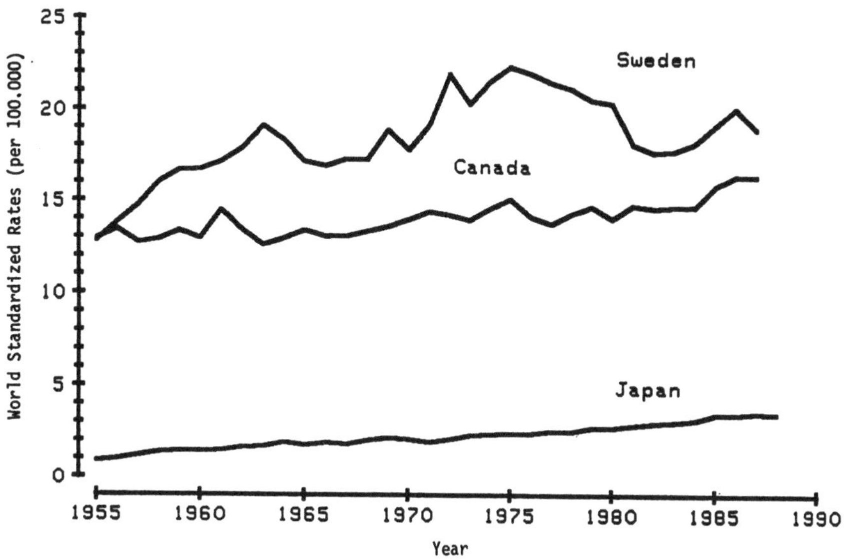

Fig. 3. Age-standardised mortality rates from prostate cancer in Sweden, Japan and Canada 1955-1988

rates are observed in countries of South-East Asia [3]. It should be noted that prostatic cancer rates are also high in blacks in Africa, being of the same order as the rates in Western Europe [3,6,7].

The highest mortality rates for prostatic cancer are to be found in Carribean countries - St. Vincent and Grenadines and Martinique, unfortunately countries from which no incidence statistics are available [4]. Mortality rates are also high in Sweden and Norway while in North America and Europe rates are lower (Fig. 2). Once more, the lowest levels of mortality for prostatic cancer are reported from oriental countries [4].

Figure 3 presents the time trends in mortality rates from prostate cancer in Canada, Japan and Sweden: these 3 countries chosen covering the range of prostate cancer variation. The mortality rate is increasing in all 3 countries since 1955. In 1988, however, prostate cancer comprised 2.49% of all cancer deaths among men in Japan, with the corresponding figure for Canada being 10.64% and for Sweden 17.73%. This emphasises the importance of prostate cancer as a public health problem. When the age-specific mortality rates for these same countries are examined by birth cohort, it is suggestive that rates are beginning to fall in the younger cohorts in Japan (Fig. 4) and Canada (Fig. 5) but this drop is not yet apparent in Sweden (Fig. 6).

Prostatic cancer can be subdivided into 3 distinct categories: clinical prostatic cancer, which produces symptoms and, as the name implies, can be diagnosed clinically; occult cancer, which produces clinically overt met-

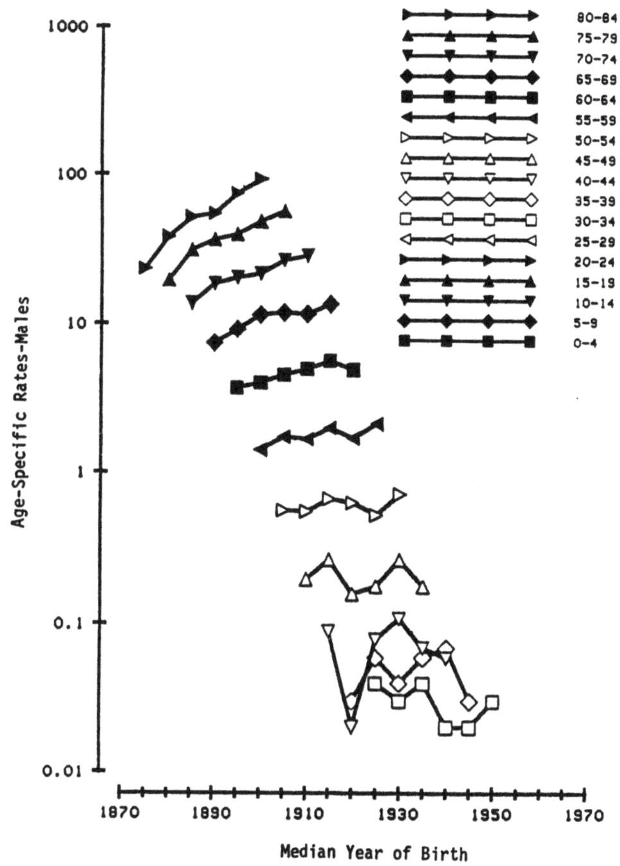

Fig. 4. Mortality from prostate cancer in Japan by birth cohort 1955-1988

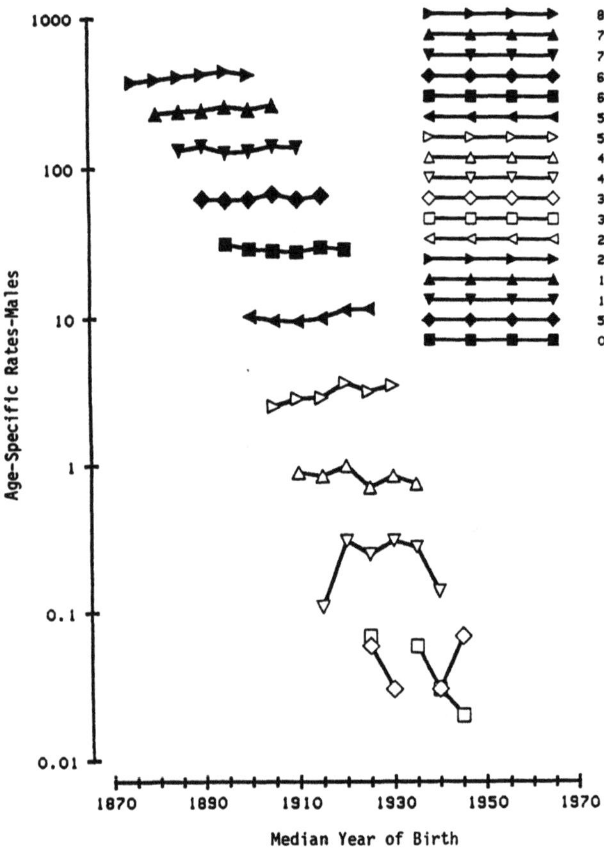

Fig. 5. Mortality from prostate cancer in Canada by birth cohort 1955-1988

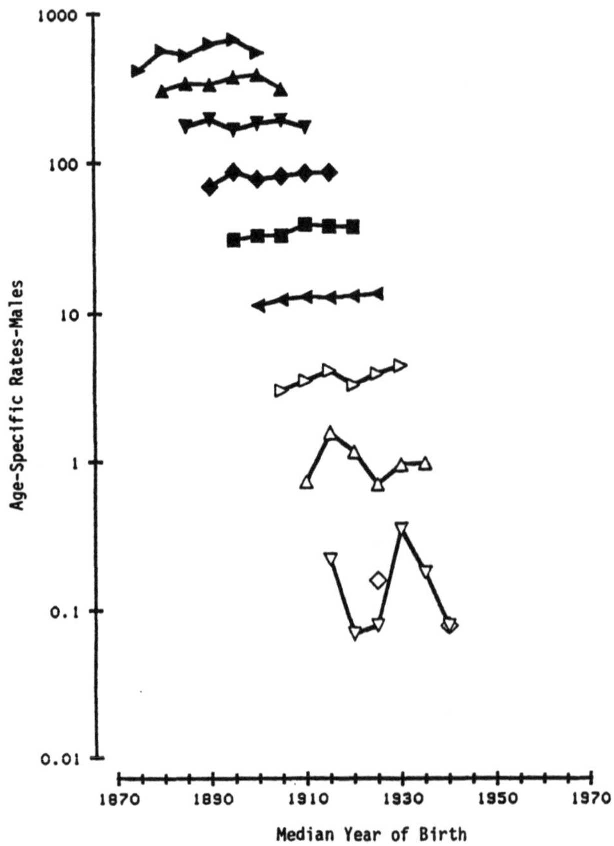

Fig. 6. Mortality from prostate cancer in Sweden by birth cohort 1955-1988

astasis while the primary lesion remains insignificant in size or hidden; latent cancer, which is clinically unrecognizable and is usually an incidental finding at prostatectomy or autopsy.

The frequency of latent carcinoma, unlike the frequency of clinical cancer, does not appear to vary internationally or among different ethnic groups. Several autopsy studies have reported a similar prevalence of small, non-invasive latent carcinoma in populations with contrasting incidence rates of clinically overt prostatic cancer [8-12]. The available statistics on prostatic cancer incidence and mortality are based on the sum of clinically diagnosed carcinomas and those latent tumours found unexpectedly at prostatectomy or autopsy. The proportion of cases of latent carcinoma among all prostatic cancer cases obviously depends on its detection rate and varies from country to country, casting uncertainty on the comparability of prostatic cancer statistics from different areas [2].

Zaridze and Boyle [4] noted the importance of the observation that the prevalence of small latent carcinomas is about 20% in men aged 45 years and remains unchanged with increasing age [9], while the incidence of clinical prostatic cancer increases rapidly with increasing age and that this increase is more rapid than for any other form of cancer [13].

Migrant studies have demonstrated that migrants from low- to high-incidence areas acquire a higher risk for prostatic cancer [14-16], with an increase in risk already apparent in the first generation of migrants from Japan and China. Haenszel [14] has shown that migrants from Ireland, Norway, Canada and Sweden have higher prostatic cancer rates than other United States whites, while migrants from Austria, Poland, USSR and Italy show lower rates.

The cancer experience of special population groups, whose lifestyle habits distinguish them from the general population and also from the nearby population, is of great interest in relation to cancer sites in which certain lifestyle factors are claimed to be of aetiological importance. The most studied of such groups are Seventh-Day Adventists and Mormons, whose cancer and cardiovascular disease experience and lifestyle pattern have been the subject of rigorous studies.

In general, currently available evidence on cancer among Seventh-Day Adventists and Mormons is consistent with the hypothesis that one or more components of the typical Adventists' and Mormons' lifestyle account for a large proportion of their reduced risk of cancer. However, the rates for prostatic cancer in Seventh-Day Adventists do not differ from those in control populations [17], while the incidence of prostatic cancer is higher among Mormons than among non-Mormons [18].

The descriptive epidemiology of prostate cancer can be summarised as providing compelling evidence that prostate cancer may be preventable. Different populations around the world experience different levels of prostate cancer and these levels change systematically with time. When migration takes place, migrant groups quickly acquire the prostate cancer pattern of their new home. Furthermore, groups of individuals whose lifestyle differentiates themselves from other members of the same community experience different prostate cancer levels. While the data on blacks in Africa and the United States provide some evidence of a genetic component to prostate cancer risk, it is clear that lifestyle comprises a large fraction of the causes of prostate cancer.

Suspected Aetiological Factors

Hormones

It is not the purpose of this chapter to give a detailed review of endocrinological factors in the aetiology of cancer of the prostate: this will be discussed in some of the following chapters in this volume. In this chapter brief mention only will be made with some important references quoted and it can be easily summarised. In research directed to the search for endocrine or biochemical factors that could be implicated in prostate carcinogenesis, determination of steroid and peptide hormone concentrations in plasma of patients with the disease has failed to consistently identify any endocrine disturbance, or any difference from the normal asymptomatic male which could lead to a greater understanding of prostate cancer aetiology [19].

Sex hormones have been implicated in the aetiology of cancer of the prostate, primarily on the basis that the growth and development of this organ requires the presence of sex hormones. The hormonal hypothesis in the aetiology of prostatic cancer is supported by the discovery of steroid hormone receptors in prostatic carcinoma [20], by the success of oestrogen treatment of prostatic cancer patients [21] and, finally, by the fact that it was possible to induce prostatic carcinoma in experimental animals by prolonged administration of male sex hormones [22]. In addition, it has been shown that the levels of testosterone and dihydrotestosterone are higher in neoplastic prostatic tissue than in the normal prostatic gland, as is the uptake of testosterone and its conversion to its metabolite dihydrotestosterone. The level of testosterone in neoplastic tissue has been found to be higher than in the hyperplastic prostate while, conversely, the levels of dihydrotestosterone were higher in the hyperplastic prostatic gland [23-25].

However, the hormonal hypothesis in the development of prostatic cancer has received only equivocal support from epidemiological studies and clinical observations. Evidence from correlation studies does not clearly indicate differences in hormone profiles of high- and low-risk populations [26-28]. The latter study has, however, shown a difference in plasma levels of oestradiol, oestrone and dihydrotestosterone between North American whites and blacks and South African blacks; levels of the first two hormones were higher in South Africans, while the level of the latter hormone was higher in North America. No case-control study published to date has compared levels of hormones among cases and controls. The results of clinical observation studies, in which comparisons are made between serum levels of different hormones among patients with prostatic cancer and

healthy controls, are conflicting and difficult to interpret [29-39].
More consistent results have been obtained for serum levels of prolactin: for example, in studies of serum prolactin, 3 studies found prolactin levels to be higher in patients with prostatic cancer [31,38,39]; 2 studies showed higher levels in patients with prostatic cancer than in patients with benign prostatic hyperplasia [30,35], while only 2 studies did not find any difference in levels of this hormone between patients with prostatic cancer, benign prostatic hyperplasia and/or healthy controls [33,36]. Results obtained from studies of other hormones, especially testosterone and dihydrotestosterone, are not convincing because of the lack of consistency of their results [29-32,34,37,39] (Table 2).
In the majority of the above studies, the levels of total testosterone and dihydrotestosterone were measured. The total plasma testosterone and dihydrotestosterone do not, however, reflect levels of the biologically active free fraction not bound to serum hormone binding globulin (SHBG) of these hormones and this could be one of the explanations for the inconsistency of the results. In addition, in all these studies control subjects were not matched individually with prostatic cancer patients, the age distribution of the control group was not always comparable with that of the group of patients, and the numbers of the study subjects were very small.
A further study has suggested that the levels of steroid hormones in the prostatic fluid of prostatic cancer patients and controls are different, the values of oestradiol and prolactin being high in prostate cancer patients [40].

Sexual Activity and Marital Status

Sexual activity, which is merely an indicator or indirect measure of hormonal status, has been related to the occurrence of prostatic cancer [41,42]. Prostatic cancer patients seem to have a greater sexual drive than controls, but are less sexually active. According to Rotkin [44], prostatic cancer patients experience both puberty and first intercourse at a later age than controls.
Prostatic cancer mortality rates are associated with marital status, increasing in the following order: single, married, widowed, divorced [43,44]. It has also been suggested that among married men the risk of prostatic cancer is higher in those with children than among those without children [45].
The result of case-control studies in general show the same pattern. Steele et al. [46] found that among prostatic cancer patients there was a significantly lower proportion of single men than in the control group. In other studies, prostatic cancer patients had significantly more children than controls [26,46,48]. However, these associations with marital status are more difficult to interpret today than previously with regard to their interpretation vis-a-vis sexual drive and sexual activity due to changes in Society's attitudes.

Diet

The hypothesis relating prostatic cancer to a high-fat diet, through possible influence on hormone metabolism, has arisen from observation of the international distribution of prostatic cancer [26,49]. Several correlation studies report a positive correlation between prostatic cancer frequency and a high-fat intake [49-53] and also with the frequency of other diet-related cancers such as colorectal and breast cancer [49,51,54]. In addition, there is limited evidence to suggest that diet influences the hormonal profile of men [28].
Hypotheses relating prostatic cancer risk to a high-fat diet, through a possible influence on hormone metabolism, have arisen through observation of the international distribution of prostate cancer occurrence and per capita fat intake [4]. Recent interest has focused on 3 aspects of diet: animal fat intake, beta-carotene intake and milk consumption.
Schuman et al. [55] reported a case-control study of 223 cases in Minnesota, USA, and found an increased risk (odds ratio (OR) =2.45) associated with infrequent consumption of carrots and an increased risk (OR=1.68) for frequent consumption of ice-cream. Graham et al. [56], in a study based on 260 cases, found an increased risk (OR=3.0) for high animal fat consumption. The same study found an increased risk (OR=1.8) associated with frequent consumption of vitamin A rich foods among men aged over 70.

Table 2. Summary of results of measurements of serum hormone levels in patients with prostatic cancer, patients with benign prostatic hyperplasia, and healthy persons

	Habib et al. [29]	Harper et al. [30]	Bartsch et al. [31]	Hammond et al. [33]	Hammond et al. [32]	Ghanadian et al. [34]	Griffiths et al. [35]	Jacobi et al. [36]	Jackson et al. [37]		Rolandi et al. [38]	Saroff et al. [39]
									USA	Nigeria		
Testosterone	(0)	(0)	(-)		(0)	(+)			(+)	(-)		(-)
DHT	(0)		(-)		(+)	(0)						(++)
Androsterone					(0)							
Androstenedione	(0)	(0)			(0)							
Oestradiol		(0)	(0)		(0)							
Oestron			(0)						(+)	(0)		
FSH		(0)	(0)	(0)							(0)	
LH		(0)	(+)	(+)							(0)	
Prolactin		(++)	(+)	(0)			(++)	(0)			(+)	(+)

(0) no difference
(+) higher in PC patients than in controls
(++) higher in PC patients than in BPH patients
(-) lower in PC patients than in controls

Snowdon, Phillips and Choi [57] examined 247 prostate cancers which occurred in a prospective study of Seventh-Day Adventists. They found no effect of intake of fruits and vegetables. However, they found a significantly increased risk (OR=2.4) associated with frequent milk consumption and a significant risk (OR=3.6) associated with a heavy intake of milk, cheese, eggs and meat. Heshmat et al. [58], reporting a case-control study of 181 cases, found that intake of vitamin A from plant and animal sources was higher in cases than in controls. They also found that cases consumed significantly greater amounts of fats than controls.

Hirayama [59] reported findings from a cohort study conducted in Japan which yielded 183 prostate cancer cases. He reported a reduced risk of death associated with frequent consumption of green and yellow vegetables in men aged less than 75 years. However, he found the reverse situation, i.e., a positive association, in men aged over 75. These results are difficult to reconcile at present. No data regarding fats were reported.

Talamini et al. [60] reported a case-control study from Northern Italy based on 166 cases. They reported a non-significant increased risk (OR=1.2) for men who consumed green vegetables 5 or more times per week. Prostate cancer risk was increased by frequent weekly consumption (5+ times) of milk and dairy products (OR=2.5) and meat (OR=1.7). Ross et al. [61] reported a case-control study of prostate cancer with 142 cases interviewed. In those with a high-fat diet, an increased risk (OR=2.0) was found to be associated with low beta-carotene intake. Significant risks were found for high fat intake among black subjects with a trend in risk apparent among whites.

Ohno et al. [62] found no association with dietary fat intake in their case-control study but among men aged over 70, they found an increased risk (OR=2.9) associated with low beta-carotene intake. By contrast, Kolonel, Yoshizawa and Hankin [63] based on a larger case-control study (452 cases) found an increased risk (OR=1.6) associated with higher levels of dietary beta-carotene intake among men aged over 70. They also found an increased risk (OR=1.7) associated with high usual consumption of saturated fat among men aged over 70.

Mettlin et al. [64] reported findings from a case-control study of 371 cases in Buffalo, New York. A decreased risk for high beta-carotene intake was found for both younger (less than 69) men (OR=0.3 in highest quintile) but not among older (70+) men (OR=1.0 in highest quintile). This study also found a trend toward increased risk for intake of fat from meats and a significantly increased risk associated with preference for whole milk (OR=1.9). Mills et al. [65] reported follow-up on a Seventh-Day Adventist cohort which yielded 180 cases of prostate cancer. Increasing consumption of fruits was associated with a significantly decreased risk and a suggestive positive association with animal product consumption did not persist after adjustment.

The situation vis-à-vis these findings is difficult to summarise concisely. Fat intake probably increases the risk of prostate cancer and while milk consumption is also apparently associated it has not been shown to be independent of intake of fat. The association with vegetable intake is very confusing: some studies are positive, some negative and a smaller number are null. It is clear, however, that there are dietary determinants of prostate cancer risk but their precise nature remains to be identified in a variety of populations in a variety of study designs.

The suggestion from some studies that increased beta-carotene/vitamin A/vegetable intake increases the risk of prostate cancer deserves to be taken seriously, particularly in view of its possible protective role and use as a chemoprevention agent against many common forms of cancer. It has been shown that vitamin A can enhance carcinogenesis in some animal models [66]. With specific regard to the prostate, it has been shown that vitamin A may influence the synthesis of testosterone and that vitamin A has metabolic interactions with zinc (which may itself be a prostate cancer risk factor (see below)). Further, vitamin A can enhance proliferation of prostatic epithelial cells [67] and hence progress on occult tumours. However, support for a possible protective effect of vitamin A is supported by laboratory findings which have shown that vitamin A and synthetic retinoids inhibit and reverse carcinogen-induced hyperplastic and anaplastic lesions in mouse prostate organ cultures [68].

In studies which have examined the effect of dietary intake of trace elements on the frequency of cancer, a direct correlation has been established between estimated zinc and cadmium intake and mortality from prostatic cancer, as well as cancer of the large bowel, breast, uterus and skin. This finding is suggested not to represent the direct effect of increased zinc and cadmium intake but rather to be an indirect effect of zinc and cadmium on cancer risk by their antagonism with selenium, which was found to be inversely correlated with mortality from the above cancers [69]. There is evidence that levels of zinc in neoplastic prostatic tissue are significantly lower than in normal prostatic gland, whereas in gland with benign prostatic hyperplasia, levels of zinc are significantly elevated [70-72]. The suggestion on the possible role of cadmium in prostatic carcinogenesis is based on the ability of cadmium to modify the capacity of the prostate to take up zinc [73].

The currently available epidemiological evidence by no means provides definitive evidence that prostate cancer risk is increased by increased intake of vitamin A or beta-carotene rich foods or supplements. It merely highlights an area of possible concern in epidemiology, particularly when making dietary recommendations to bring about cancer prevention.

Body Mass Index

In the American Cancer Society cohort, overweight males were shown to have a 30 % increased prostate cancer mortality compared to men within 10% of their "ideal" weight [74]. Among Seventh-Day Adventists, the risk of fatal prostate cancer was 2.5-fold elevated among overweight men [57]. Two case-control studies were inconclusive [26,55]. More recently, Talamini et al. found a substantial dose-response gradient in a case-control study in Northern Italy [60]. With the risk set to 1.0 in the lowest tertile of Body Mass Index (kg per metre squared), the risk rose to 2.3 (95% C.I. (2.1,4.8)) in the second tertile and to 4.4 (1.9,9.9) in the highest: the trend was highly significant ($p<.001$).

Given these findings and the association between energy intake and increased weight, it is important to have information on dietary intake of vitamin A and beta-carotene adjusted for total energy intake. As Willett [75] has pointed out, people who have high energy intakes generally eat more of everything: thus they will apparently have an increased carotene/vitamin A intake due to what could be an artefact. It is essential to look at the micronutrients associated with prostate cancer risk after adjustment for estimated energy intake: this does not appear to have been done to date.

Occupation

In experimental conditions, several cadmium compounds have been reported to be carcinogenic [76], although administration of cadmium components failed to produce any changes in the prostate gland of experimental animals [77,78]. The results of cohort studies suggest an increased risk of prostatic cancer among those who were exposed to cadmium oxide [79,80]. A case-control study in which exposure to dietary sources of cadmium was related to prostatic cancer risk produced negative results [81].

In cohort studies of rubber workers, an excess of prostatic cancer death was observed [82-84]. In one of these studies, an excess of prostatic cancer deaths was claimed to be the result of exposure to cadmium [82]. However, this hypothesis was subsequently rejected [85]. An attempt to find a specific work experience with specific exposure in the rubber industry has not yet been successful.

While several studies have demonstrated an increased risk of prostate cancer among farmers and agriculture workers [86,87], a recent study from New Zealand did not provide support for this association [88]. A feature of studies of occupation and prostate cancer has been that findings in one are not replicated in the others and a new set of occupations are found to be associated with higher risk (see discussion in [87]).

Genetic Factors

Prostate cancer was found to be significantly more frequent in the male relatives of index patients than in controls [46,89]. Furthermore, the high levels reported in blacks worldwide -

Africa, the Carribean and North America, suggest a possible independent genetic component to the risk of this disease.

Sexually Transmitted Infection

There is evidence from experimental studies that certain tumour-associated viruses isolated from a human prostate carcinoma (Herpes virus 2, Simian virus 40, and cytomegalovirus) are able to induce oncogenic transformation of hamster embryo cells [90-92]. A number of studies have demonstrated the presence of virus-like particles in tissue removed from patients with prostatic cancer [93] or have shown increased antibody titres in such patients [94].

In several case-control studies, a higher proportion of cases than controls reported a previous history of venereal disease [42,46,89]. (This may also reflect the tendency, discussed above, of prostatic cancer cases to have a greater sexual drive.) Some studies have observed an increase in breast and cervical cancer among wives of men with prostatic cancer [95] but others failed to confirm the previous findings [96].

Benign Prostatic Hyperplasia

The relationship between benign prostatic hyperplasia and prostatic cancer remains controversial [4]. The 2 most frequently quoted studies on the relationship between benign prostatic hyperplasia and prostatic cancer have produced contrasting results [48,97]. In the second study, both prospective and retrospective approaches were used. The results obtained from the prospective study demonstrate a relative risk of prostatic cancer 3.7 times greater among benign prostatic hyperplasia patients, and indicate that prostatectomy produces a considerable reduction in subsequent cancer risk. The retrospective study of patients with prostate cancer and controls admitted with benign prostatic hyperplasia has shown a relative risk of 5.1 for the prostatic cancer group. These findings are at variance with the results of a prospective study of patients who had subtotal prostatectomy and controls, in which the relative risk of prostatic cancer in the benign prostatic hyperplasia group was estimated to be 0.9 [48]. Furthermore, it is generally accepted that carcinoma arises in the outer part of the prostate, while benign prostatic hyperplasia is more often found in the inner part of the gland [9,98,99].

Discussion

The association of the hormonal profile of men with diet and, most probably, diet-associated differences in the hormonal milieu of populations at different risk of prostatic cancer, suggests that diet determines the risk of prostatic cancer through its influence on sex hormone metabolism. As has been shown above, prostatic cancer is a disease of old age, and its incidence increases rapidly with age, suggesting that the hormonal status of elderly men and the changes which occur with advancing age should be of importance in the aetiology of prostatic cancer.

Carcinogenesis is recognised as a multistage process which results from a complex interaction of multiple factors. There are two clearly defined stages in the natural history of prostatic cancer. The end point of the first stage of carcinogenesis in the prostate is the development of a latent cancer (small, focal, clinically unrecognizable tumour), while the second stage evolves into an invasive clinically overt tumour. While little is known about the factors involved in the first stage of prostatic carcinogenesis, the second stage, which is associated with tumour growth, promotion and progression, is, most probably, related aetiologically to environmental factors prevalent in the high-risk populations, frequently defined as "lifestyle" factors.

Some epidemiological observations, however, are compatible with the hypothesis that there is a genetic component in the aetiology of prostatic cancer. First of all, cancer of the prostate was found more frequently in the male relatives of index patients than in controls [35,36]. Secondly, the incidence of prostatic cancer has been reported to be high not only among North American blacks, who consume a Western diet, but also in blacks living in Africa [32,6,7], whose diet is mainly vegetarian. Thirdly, according to the most recent incidence statistics [3], prostatic cancer incidence among Japanese and Chinese in most areas of the United States is still less than half that of white Americans, while their rates for colorectal cancer (cancer with high-fat diet related aetiology) are of the same order as those of white and black Americans. The above suggests either that Chinese and Japanese may be less susceptible to prostatic cancer than blacks and/or Caucasians, or that there are some unknown exogenous factors to which the latter but not the former ethnic groups are exposed.

Where do we stand currently (1990) with the epidemiology of prostatic cancer? The disease is increasing in incidence in many parts of the world at differing disease risks and we do not understand which risk factor(s) are driving these spatial and temporal differences. The findings from aetiological studies are inconsistent in regards to the likely important variables: these are probably dietary and hormonal in origin but it is not clear which one is the "true" risk factor. There is some agreement that neither cigarette smoking nor alcohol drinking are risk factors for prostate cancer. From the available evidence, it is "probable" that a diet high in fat and milk increases the risk of prostate cancer. It is difficult to ignore the various suggestions that beta-carotene/ vitamin A rich diets could be associated with an increased risk of prostate cancer. This is particularly true at a time when these micronutrients are being proposed for cancer prevention strategies. Finally, it is difficult to escape the feeling that prostatic cancer has not attracted the interest from epidemiologists that its numerical importance deserves: the reviewer is left somewhat frustrated by the low number of studies and the relative absence of large numbers of good-quality studies. The problem is much too important to ignore.

REFERENCES

1 Parkin DM, Laara E and Muir CS: Estimates of the worldwide frequency of sixteen major cancers in 1980. Int J Cancer 1988 (41):184-197

2 Zaridze DG, Boyle P and Smans M: Trends in prostatic cancer. Int J Cancer 1984 (33):223-230

3 MuirCS, Waterhouse JAH, Mack T, Powell J, Whelan S (eds) Cancer Incidence in Five Continents Vol V IARC Scientific Publication No 88, International Agency for Research on Cancer, Lyon

4 Zaridze DG and Boyle P: Cancer of the prostate: epidemiology and etiology. Br J Urol 1987 (59):493-503

5 HakulinenT, Andersen AA, Malker B, Pukkula E, Schou G and Tulinius H: Trends in cancer incidence in the Nordic Countries. Acta Pathol Microbiol Immunol Scand 1986 (94 Suppl 228)

6 Waterhouse JAH, Muir CS, Correa P and Powell J (eds). Cancer Incidence in Five Continents Vol III. IARC Scientific Publication No 15. International Agency for Research on Cancer, Lyon 1976

7 Waterhouse JAH, Muir CS, Shanmugaratnam K and Powell J eds: Cancer Incidence in Five Continents Vol IV. IARC Scientific Publication No 42. International Agency for Research on Cancer, Lyon 1982

8 Akazaki K and Stemmerman GN: Comparative study of latent carcinoma of the prostate among Japanese in Japan and Hawaii. JNCI 1973 (50):1137-1144

9 Breslow N, Chan CE, Dhom G, Drury RAB, Franks LM, Gellei B, Lee YS, Lundberg S, Sparke B, Sternby NH and Tulinius H: Latent carcinoma of prostate at autopsy in seven areas. Int J Cancer 1977 (20):680-688

10 Guileyardo JM, Johnson WD, Welsh RA, Akazaki K and Correa P: Prevalence of latent prostate carcinoma in two U.S. populations. JNCI 1980 (65):311-316

11 Correa P and London JL: Time trends in the Americas. In: Magnus K (ed) Trends in Cancer Incidence, Causes and Practical Implications. Part 7: Cancer of the Prostate. A publication of the International Union Against Cancer and the Norwegian Cancer Society. Hemisphere Publishing Corporation, Washington DC 1982 pp 335-345

12 Yatani R, Chigusa K, Akazaki K, Stemmermann GN, Welsh RA and Correa P: Geographic pathology of latent prostatic carcinoma. Int J Cancer 1982 (29):611-616

13 Cook PJ, Doll R and Fellingham SA: A mathematical model for the age distribution of cancer in man. Int J Cancer 1969 (4):93-112

14 Haenszel W: Cancer mortality among the foreign-born in the United States. JNCI 1961 (26):37-132

15 Haenszel W and Kurihara M: Studies of Japanese migrants. I. Mortality from cancer and other diseases among Japanese in the United States. JNCI 1968 (40):43-68

16 King H and Haenszel W: Cancer mortality among foreign- and native-born Chinese in the United States. J Chron Dis 1968 (26):623-646

17 Phillips RL, Kuzma JW and Lotz TM: Cancer mortality among comparable members versus non-members of the Seventh-Day Adventist Church. In: Cairns J, Lyon JL and Skolnick M (eds) Cancer Incidence in Defined Populations. Banbury Report 4. Cold Spring Harbor Laboratory, New York 1980 pp 93-108

18 Lyon JL, Gardner JW and West DW: Cancer risk and life-style: cancer among Mormons from 1967-1975. In: Cairns J, Lyon JL and Skolnick M (eds) Cancer Incidence in Defined Populations. Banbury Report 4. Cold Spring Harbor Laboratory, New York 1980 pp 3-30

19 Griffiths K et al:. Endocrine factors in the initiation, diagnosis and treatment of prostatic cancer. In: Voight KD and Knabbec C (eds) Endocrine Dependent Tumours. Raven Press, New York 1990

20 Murphy LJT: The prostate. In: The History of Urology. Charles C Thomas, Springfield 1972 pp 378-452

21 Mainwaring IP: Steroid receptors and the regulation of transcriptional events in the prostate. In: Coffey DS and Isaacs JT (eds) Prostatic Cancer: A Series of Workshops on the Biology of Human Cancer. UICC Technical Report Series, Vol 48, Report No 9, pp 126-130. International Union against Cancer, Geneva 1979

22 Noble KL: The development of prostate adenocarcinoma in the Nb rat following prolonged sex hormone administration. Cancer Res 1977 (37):1929-1233

23 Habib FK, Lee IR, Stitch SR and Smith PH: Androgen levels in the plasma and prostatic tissues of patients with benign hypertrophy and carcinoma of the prostate. J Endocrinol 1976 (71):99-107

24 Geller J, Albert J, de la Vega D, Loza D and Stoeltzing W (1978). Dihydrotestosterone concentration in prostate cancer tissue as a predictor of tumor differentiation and hormonal dependency. Cancer Res 1978 (38):4349-4352

25 Krieg M, Bartsch W and Voigt KD: Binding, metabolism and tissue level of androgens in human prostatic carcinoma, benign prostatic hyperplasia and normal prostate. Exerpta Medica International Congresses Series 1980 (494):102-104

26 Wynder EL, Mabuchi K and Whitmore WF: Epidemiology of cancer of the prostate. Cancer 1971 (28):344-360
27 Hill P, Wynder EL, Garbaczewski L, Garnes H and Walker ARP: Diet and urinary steroids in black and white North American men and black South African men. Cancer Res 1979 (39):5101-5105
28 Hill P, Wynder EL, Garnes H and Walker ARP: Environmental factors, hormone status and prostatic cancer. Preventive Med 1980 (9):657-666
29 Habib FK and Stitch SR: Hormones, elderly testes and carcinoma of the prostate. Br Med J 1975 (4):650
30 Harper ME, Peeling WB, Cowley T, Brownsey BG, Phillips MEA, Groom G, Fahmy DR and Griffiths K: Plasma steroid and protein hormone concentrations in patients with prostatic carcinoma, before and during oestrogen therapy. Acta Endocrinologica 1976 (81):409-426
31 Bartsch W, Steins P and Becker H: Hormone blood levels in patients with prostatic carcinoma and their relation to the type of carcinoma growth differentiation. Eur Urology 1977 (7):129-135
32 Hammond GL: Endogenous steroid levels in the human prostate from birth to old age: a comparison of normal and diseased tissues. J Endocrinol 1978 (78):7-19
33 Hammond GL, Kontturi M, Määttälä P, Puukka M and Vhiko R: Serum FSH, LH and prolactin in normal males and patients with prostatic diseases. Clin Endocrinol 1977 (7):129-135
34 Ghanadian R, Puah CM and O'Donoghue EPN: Serum testosterone and dihydrotestosterone in carcinoma of the prostate. Br J Cancer 1979 (39):696-699
35 Griffiths K, Peeling WB, Groom GU, Sibley PE and Harper ME: Protein hormones and prostatic cancer. Progr Cancer ResTher 1980 (144):185-192
36 Jacobi GH, Rathgen GH and Altwein JE: Serum prolactin and tumors of the prostate: unchanged basal levels and lack of correlation to serum testosterone. J Endocrinol Invest 1980 (3):15-18
37 Jackson MA, Kovi J, Heshmat MY, Jones GW, Rao MS and Ahlwalia BS: Characterization of prostatic carcinoma among blacks: a comparison between a low-incidence area, Ibadan, Nigeria, and a high-incidence area, Washington, DC. Prostate 1980 (1):185-205
38 Rolandi E, Pescatore D, Milesi GM, Giberti C, Sannia A and Barreca T: Evaluation of LH, FSH, TSH, Prl and GH secretion in patients suffering from prostatic neoplasma. Acta Endocrinologica 1980 (95):23-26
39 Saroff J, Kirdani Y, Ming Chu T, Wajsman Z and Murphy GP: Measurements of prolactin and androgens in patients with prostatic diseases. Oncology 1980 (37):46-52
40 Wynder EL, Laakso K, Sotaranta M and Rose DP: Metabolic epidemiology of prostatic cancer. Prostate 1984 (5):47-53
41 Rotkin ID: Studies in the epidemiology of prostatic cancer: Expanded sampling. Cancer Treat Rep 1977 (61):173-180
42 Schuman LM, Mandel J, Blackard C, Bauer H, Scarlett J and McHugh R: Epidemiologic study of prostatic cancer: Preliminary report. Cancer Treat Rep 1977 (61):181-186
43 King M, Diamond E and Lilienfeld AM: Some epidemiological aspects of cancer of the prostate. J Chron Dis 1963 (16):117-153
44 Lilienfeld AM, Levin ML and Kessler II: Cancer in the United States. American Public Health Association Monograph. Harvard University Press, Cambridge MA 1972
45 Lancaster HO: The mortality in Australia from cancer peculiar to the male. Med J Australia 1972 (2):41-44
46 Steele R, Lees REM, Kraus AS and Rao C: Sexual factors in the epidemiology of cancer of the prostate. J Chron Dis 1971 (24):29-37
47 Greenwald P, Damon A, Kirmss V and Polan AK: Physical and demographic features of men before developing cancer of the prostate. JNCI 1974 (53):341-346
48 Armenian HK, Lilienfeld AM, Diamond EL and Bross IDJ: Epidemiologic characteristics of patients with prostate neoplasms. Am J Epidemiol 1975 (102):47-54
49 Berg JW: Can nutrition explain the pattern of international epidemiology of hormone-dependent cancers? Cancer Res 1975 (35):3345-3350
50 Howell MA: Factor analysis of international cancer mortality data and per capita food consumption. Br J Cancer 1974 (29):328-336
51 Armstrong B and Doll R: Environmental factors and cancer incidence and mortality in different countries, with special reference to dietary practices. Int J Cancer 1975 (15):617-631
52 Blair A and Fraumeni JF: Geographic patterns of prostate cancer in the United States. JNCI 1978 (61):1379-1384
53 Kolonel LN, Hankin JH, Lee J, Chu SY, Nomura AMY and Hinds MW: Nutrient intakes in relation to cancer incidence in Hawaii. Br J Cancer 1981 (44):332-339
54 Burbank FA: Sequential space-time cluster analysis of cancer mortality in the United States: Etiologic implications. Am J Epidemiol 1972 (95):393-417
55 Schuman LM, Mandel J, Radke A et al: Some selected features of the epidemiology of prostatic cancer: Minneapolis- St.Paul, Minnesota case-

control study, 1976-1979. In: Magnus K (ed) Trends in Cancer Incidence, Causes and Practical Implications. Hemisphere Press, Washington DC 1982 pp 345-354

56 Graham S, Haughey B, Marshall J, Priore R, Byers T, Rzepka T, Mettling C, Pontes JE: Diet in the epidemiology of carcinoma of the prostate gland. JNCI 1983 (70):687-692

57 Snowden DA, Phillips RL and Choi W: Diet, obesity and risk of fatal prostate cancer. Am J Epidemiol 1984 (120):244-250

58 Heshmat MY, Kaul L, Kovi et al: Nutrition and prostate cancer: a case-control study. Prostate 1985 (6):7-17

59 Hirayama T: A large-scale cohort study on cancer risks by diet with special reference to the risk reducing effects of green-yellow vegetable consumption. In: Hayashi T, Nagao M and Sugimura T (eds) Diet, Nutrition and Cancer. Japan Scientific Societies Press, Tokyo 1986 pp 41-47

60 Talamini R, La Vecchia C, DeCarli A et al: Nutrition, social factors and prostatic cancer in a Northern Italian population. Br J Cancer 1986 (53):817-821

61 Ross RK, Shimizu H, Paganini-Hill A, Honda G and Henderson BE: Case-control studies of prostate cancer in blacks and whites in southern California. JNCI 1987 (78):869-874

62 Ohno Y, Yoshida O, Oishi K et al: Dietary beta-carotene and cancer of the prostate: a case-control study. Cancer Res 1988 (48):1331-1336

63 Kolonel, LN, Yoshizawa CN and Hankin JH: Diet and prostatic cancer: a case-control study in Hawaii. Am J Epidemiol 1988 (127):999-1012

64 Mettlin C, Selenskas S, Natarajan N and Huben R: Beta-carotene and animal fats and their relationship to prostate cancer risk: a case-control study. Cancer 1989 (64):605-612

65 Mills PK, Beeson WL, Phillips RL and Fraser GE: Cohort study of diet, lifestyle and prostate cancer in Adventist men. Cancer 1989 (64):598-604

66 Welsch CW, Goodrich-Smith M, Brown CK Crowe N: Enhancement by retinyl acetate of hormone-induced mammary tumorigenesis in female GR/A mice. JNCI 1981 (67):935-948

67 Chaproniere P, Webber W: Dexamethozone and retinyl acetate work similarly to inhibit and stimulate EGF- or insulin-induced proliferation of prostatic epithelium. J Cell Physiol 1985 (122):249-253

68 Chopra DP and Wilkoff LJ: Effects of carcinogens and retinoids on prostatic explants. Clin Andrology 1981 (6):166-174

69 Schrauzer GN, White DA and Schneider CJ: Cancer mortality correlation studies - III. Statistical associations with dietary selenium intakes. Bioinorganic Chemistry 1977 (7):23-34

70 Schrodt GR, Hall T and Whitmore WR: The concentration of zinc in diseased human prostate gland. Cancer 1964 (17):1555-1556

71 Gyorkey F, Min KW, Huff JA and Gyorkey P: Zinc and magnesium in human prostate - normal, hypertrophic and neoplastic. Cancer Res 1967 (27):1348-1353

72 Dhar, NK, Goel TC, Dube PC, Chowdhury AR and Kar AB: Distribution and concentration of zinc in the subcellular fractions of benign hyperplastic and malignant neoplastic human prostate. Exp Mol Pathol 1973 (19):139-142

73 Gunn SA, Gould TC and Anderson WAD: Competition of cadmium for zinc in rat testis and dorsolateral prostate. Acta Endocrinologica 1961 (37):24-30

74 Lew EA and Garfinkel L: Variations in mortality by weight among 750,000 men and women. J Chron Dis 1979 (32):563-576

75 Willett WC: Nutritional Epidemiology. Oxford University Press, New York 1990

76 International Agency for Research on Cancer: Some Inorganic and Organometallic Compounds. IARC Monograph on the Evaluation of the Carcinogenic Risk of Chemicals to Humans, Vol 2. International Agency for Research on Cancer, Lyon 1973

77 Levy LS and Clack J: Further studies on the effect of cadmium on the prostate gland. I. Absence of prostatic changes in rats given oral cadmium sulphate for two years. Ann Occup Hygiene 1975 (17):205-211

78 Levy LS, Clack J and Roe FJC (1975). Further studies on the effect of cadmium on the prostate gland. II. Absence of prostatic changes in mice given oral cadmium sulphate for eighteen months. Ann Occup Hygiene 1975 (17):213-220

79 Kipling MD and Waterhouse JAH: Cadmium and prostatic carcinoma. Lancet 1967 (i):730-731

80 Holden J: Cadmium toxicology. [mLancet 1969 (ii)57

81 Kolonel LN and Winkelstein W: Cadmium and prostatic carcinoma. Lancet 1977 (ii):566-567

82 McMichael AJ, Spirtas R, Gamble JF and Tousey PM: Mortality among rubber workers: Relationship to specific jobs. J Occup Med 1976 (18):178-185

83 Monson RJ and Nakano KK: Mortality among rubber workers. I. White male union employees in Akron, Ohio. Am J Epidemiol 1976 (103):284-296

84 Andjelkovic D, Taulbee J, Symons M and Williams T: Mortality of rubber workers with reference to work experience. J Occup Med 1977 (19):397-405

85 Goldsmith DF, Smith AH and McMichael AJ: A case-control study of prostate cancer within a cohort of

rubber and tire workers. J Occup Med 1980 (22):533-401
86 McDonald E: Natural history of prostate cancer. Proc Third National Cancer Conference. Lippincott, Philadelphia 1957
87 Blair A, Malker H, Kantor KP, et al: Cancer among farmers: a review. Scand J W Environ Health 1985 (11):397-407
88 Pearce NE, Sheppard RA and Fraser J: Case-control study of occupation and cancer of the prostate in New Zealand. J Epidemiol Comm Hlth 1987 (41):130-132
89 Krain LS: Some epidemiologic variables in prostatic carcinoma in California. Prev Med 1974 (3):154-159
90 Centifanto YM, Zam ZS, Kaufman HE and Drylie DM: In vitro transformation of hamster cells by herpes simplex virus type 2 from human prostatic cancer cells. Cancer Res 1975 (35):1880-1886
91 Paulson DF, Bonar RA, Sharief Y, Vergara JR, Reich C and Shah KV: Properties of prostatic cultures transformed by SV-40. Cancer Chemother Rep 1975 (59):51-55
92 Geder L, Sanford EJ, Rohner TJ and Rapp F: Cytomegalovirus and cancer of the prostate: In vitro transformation of human cells. Cancer Treat Rep 1977 (61):139-146
93 Webber MM, Stonington OG and Lehman J: Virus in prostatic epithelium of man. Urology 1973 (1):561-567
94 Ablin RJ: Serum antibody in patients with prostatic cancer. Br J Urol 1976 (48):355-361
95 Feminella JG and Lattimer JK: An apparent increase in genital carcinomas among wives of men with prostatic cancer. Pirquet Bull Clin Med 1973 (20):3-10
96 Greenwald P, Kirmss V and Burnett WS: Prostate cancer epidemiology. Widowhood and cancer in spouses. JNCI 1979 (62):1131-1136
97 Armenian HK, Lilienfeld AM, Diamond EL and Bross ID: Relation between benign prostatic hyperplasia and cancer of the prostate: A prospective and retrospective study. Lancet 1974 (ii):115-117
98 Franks LM: The incidence of carcinoma of prostate: an epidemiological survey. In: Grundmann E and Tulinius H (eds) Recent Results in Cancer Research 1972 (39):149-155
99 Boyle P, McGinn R, Maisonneuve P and La Vecchia C: Epidemiology of benign prostatic hyperplasia: Present knowledge and studies needed. Eur J Urol 1990 (in press)

The Molecular Biology of Prostate Cancer

Jan Trapman

Department of Pathology, Erasmus University, P.O. Box 1738, 3000 DR Rotterdam, The Netherlands

Induction and progressive growth of cancer are considered to be genetic processes. A series of mutations in different genes is believed to be necessary for development of a malignant tumour. Genetic changes can vary from a drastic damage of the genomic structure (gene amplification, chromosomal translocation, gene deletion) to a very subtle point mutation. A mutation in the gene can influence the properties of the protein product and/or its expression level.

In the case of neoplastic growth, the balance between cell proliferation and differentiation is distorted. Therefore, it was proposed already many years ago that the genes which play a role in the natural process of regulation of cell growth and differentiation are the major candidates for modification in tumour cells. Additional genetic alterations might cause invasive growth and metastasis at a later stage of tumour development.

During the last decade, our knowledge of the molecular biology of genes involved in oncogenesis has increased enormously. The literature on this subject has been discussed extensively in several review papers published in the past few years [1-7].

Especially in rodent and avian model systems, a large variety of genes involved in tumourigenesis has been detected. This group of genes has been designated oncogenes. More than 50 oncogenes have been characterised. A second category of genes, which was postulated more recently, are the tumour suppressor genes (or anti-oncogenes). Much less is known of genes and proteins which play a key role in the invasive growth and metastasis of a tumour, although in some model systems evidence has been obtained that the same genes which are associated with tumour induction are also involved in these processes.

A short review of the molecular biology of cancer is presented here, followed by the description of our current knowledge of the molecular biology of prostatic cancer. Because of the essential role of androgens in the development of the prostate gland and the importance of endocrine therapy in prostatic cancer, the molecular biology of androgen action will also be discussed.

Oncogenes and Tumourigenesis

Detection of Oncogenes

Nowadays, oncogenes can be detected by a variety of experimental approaches. Initially, however, oncogenes were discovered in correlation with RNA tumour viruses (retroviruses). The RNA genome of these viruses replicates via a double-stranded DNA intermediate. This proviral DNA can integrate in the cellular genome. Subsequently, the host cell uses its own functions to express the viral genes. Both the integration of the viral DNA in the cellular genome and the expression of specific viral genes can cause a distortion of cellular functions.

1. Many retroviruses (the so-called acute transforming viruses) carry in their genome a piece of genetic information, that was derived from a cellular gene. This mutated cellular gene is the tumourigenic part of the virus (the viral oncogene). The corresponding "normal" gene which is present in the cellular genome,

is called the cellular oncogene or proto-oncogene. The total number of oncogenes detected in this way is more than 20. Examples are *Ha-ras, src, abl, mos, myc, myb, sis, erbA, erbB, fos, jun, fms* and *fes*. Many of these genes are involved in development of sarcomas, leukaemias or lymphomas. The number of carcinomas induced by viral oncogenes is much smaller. Some retroviruses carry more than one oncogene in their genome. The combination *erbA/erbB* is a well known example of this group. The *erbB* gene by itself is already tumourigenic, in combination with *erbA* the tumours develop much more rapidly. In contrast, the *erbA* gene alone is unable to induce tumours.

2. A second group of retroviruses are the slow transforming viruses. In this case, the integration of the provirus in the genome itself directly influences the expression of a cellular gene by bringing this gene under control of the regulatory elements of the viral genome. This process is known as insertional mutagenesis. The total number of putative oncogenes detected in this way is approximately 10. The first oncogene found to be activated by insertional mutagenesis was the *c-myc* gene in chicken bursal lymphoma. Other well-known examples are the *int-1* and *int-2* genes. The structure and function of these genes is completely different, but both are involved in the development of mammary tumours in specific mouse strains.
3. Chromosomal translocations are also implicated in tumourigenesis. Due to the translocation process, (part of) an oncogene is brought under the control of the regulatory elements of a different gene, which leads to a modified expression pattern of a (mutated) gene. Examples of oncogenes located at translocation breakpoints are the *abl* gene in Chronic Myeloid Leukaemia and the *c-myc* gene in Burkitt's lymphoma in humans and plasmacytoma in mice.
4. Gene transfer experiments with DNA from (human) tumour cell lines or primary tumours resulted in the detection of transforming *ras* genes (*Ha-ras, Ki-ras* and *N-ras*) and the *neu* (*erbB2*) oncogene, which is related to the *erbB* oncogene. These genes and a limited number of other genes are able to induce morphological transformation of mouse 3T3 cells. It turned out that all *ras* genes with transforming capacity were mutated in codon 12, 13 or 61. This specific mutation pattern allows nowadays the direct screening of DNA from tumours for their presence by simple molecular biological techniques [7].
5. Amplification of oncogenes has also been correlated with tumourigenesis. Amplified oncogenes detected in this way include the *c-myc* and *N-myc* gene and the *erbB2* or *neu* gene. In this case, the overexpression of the cellular oncogene will be involved in the oncogenic process.

As can be deduced from the data presented above, several oncogenes have been detected by different methods. The *myc* oncogene is found at chromosomal translocation breakpoints and by gene amplification. In addition, it has been found as part of the genome of retroviruses, and its expression was activated by insertional mutagenesis. The *Ha-ras* and *Ki-ras* oncogenes have been detected in the genome of acute transforming retroviruses, by gene transfer experiments and by direct structural analysis of tumour cell DNA. These genes seem to be important for the growth of many types of tumours, whereas other oncogenes have been discovered in only one specific tumour.

Function of Oncogenes

The function of the protein products of oncogenes can roughly be subdivided into 4 different classes:

1. Products of oncogenes can be growth factors. The best known representative of this class is the *sis* oncogene present in the SSV (Simian Sarcoma Virus) genome. The natural counterpart of *sis* is the gene encoding one of the PDGF (Platelet-Derived Growth Factor) chains. A second example is the *int-2* oncogene, the cellular counterpart of which belongs to the family of FGF (Fibroblast Growth Factor) genes.
2. Many oncogenes code for protein kinases. In addition to enzymes which are

able to phosphorylate tyrosine-residues, also serine/threonine-specific kinases have been found among the oncogenes. One of these is the *mos* gene. Examples of tyrosine-specific kinases are the *abl*, *src*, *fes*, *fms* and *erbB* proteins. These proteins are located in the cytoplasm or at the cellular membrane. Interestingly, *erbB* turned out to be a truncated form of the EGF (Epidermal Growth Factor) receptor. The cellular counterpart of *fms* is the CSF-1 (Colony Stimulating Factor-1) receptor. So, in at least two occasions the natural function of an oncogene product is that of a growth factor receptor.

3. A third function of oncogenic proteins can be in the process of transduction of a signal from an activated (growth factor) receptor to the cell nucleus (signal transduction pathway). The *ras* oncogenes most probably fulfill such a function. They are located in the plasma membrane and are able to bind guanine nucleotides.
4. Many protein products of oncogenes are located in the cell nucleus (*myc*, *myb*, *fos*, *jun*, *p53*, *erbA*). The function of several of these proteins has clearly been established. The cellular counterpart of the *jun* protein is the transcription factor AP-1; that of *erbA* is the thyroid hormone receptor, which also is a transcription regulatory protein. In fact, *erbA* most probably has to be regarded as a tumour suppressor gene (see below). *ErbA* is able to bind to specific regulatory DNA sequences, without being functional as a transcription factor. In this way it inhibits the action of the natural thyroid hormone receptor, which directs cellular differentiation [8,9].

In conclusion, it can be stated, that oncogene products can directly interfere with many aspects of the cellular machinery. Correlations can be made between oncogenes and growth factor production (autocrine growth stimulation), growth factor receptors (growth factor independent growth), signal transduction and regulation of gene transcription. The process directly affected by a mutation in a cellular oncogene will no doubt influence a cascade of additional regulatory signals. This will ultimately lead to the uncontrolled proliferation of the tumour cell.

Oncogenes in Human Cancer

By far the most direct method to discover a (novel) oncogene is when a retrovirus is involved in the development of a specific kind of tumour (see above) or when a specific chromosomal translocation is found. However, only a very small number of human tumours is associated with a retrovirus (HTLV 1-Adult T cell leukaemia) and the number of specific chromosomal translocations described, although still increasing, is limited. In addition, many human tumours are heterogeneous and grow slowly, which complicates their characterisation. Therefore, it is an enormous task to detect (novel) genes involved in neoplastic growth in humans.

So far, approximately 10 oncogenes have consistently been found in specific human cancers. Most of them have already been described above. The best characterised of these genes are listed below.

1. Chromosomal translocation:
The *c-myc* gene is located on chromosome 8 at the translocation breakpoint t(2;8), t(8;14), or t(8,22) in Burkitt's lymphoma; the *c-abl* gene on chromosome 9 at the translocation breakpoint t(9;22) in Chronical Myeloid Leukaemia. Transforming genes at other specific breakpoints are less well characterised or not identified at all.

2. Gene amplification:
The *c-myc* gene is amplified in a high percentage of small-cell lung carcinoma and the closely related *N-myc* gene is amplified in many neuroblastomas. *ErbB2* (*neu*) is amplified in a large portion of mammary carcinomas and *erbB1* in gliomas.

3. Activated *ras* genes (point mutation in codon 12, 13 or 61) are found in about 20% of all human tumours. Most consistent are the mutations found in pancreatic carcinoma (over 90% of the tumours show a mutation in codon 12 of the *Ki-ras* gene). Other tumours with a high incidence of *ras* mutations are colon carcinoma (*Ki-ras*) and Acute Myeloid Leukaemia (*N-ras*).

Although there is strong evidence that the genes described above are involved in the growth of a particular tumour, in all cases their precise role still has to be determined.

Tumour Suppressor Genes

In addition to oncogenes, which, in an activated form, are capable of promoting cell transformation, the occurrence of a second class of genes, the tumour suppressor genes (or anti-oncogenes) has been postulated. In contrast to the oncogene, the tumour suppressor gene is deleted or inactivated by a specific mutation in the case of cell transformation. The natural function of a suppressor gene product could be the negative growth regulation of a cell or induction of a differentiation pathway. Mutations in tumour suppressor genes can be recessive. This implicates that two mutations (one in each of the two alleles) are needed before the effect of the mutation becomes manifest.

Two lines of investigation have led to the idea that loss of genetic information can be a cause of at least some steps of oncogenesis. The first observation was that upon fusion of a tumour cell with a normal cell, many of the hybrid cells showed a nontransformed phenotype. This indicates that the normal cell contributes genes to the tumour cell which impose normal growth control on the latter. The second line has evolved from the study of heritable tumours. The best known example of this group is retinoblastoma. In many cases deletions of a specific part of chromosomes 13 have been observed. It is now clearly established that chromosome 13 harbours a gene (Rb) whose function is lost in retinoblastoma cells. In the familial form of retinoblastoma, one of the mutations is inherited and already present in all cells. The second mutation in the Rb gene is induced later. The product of the Rb gene is a nuclear protein. Although the precise function of the protein has not yet been established, it is of great interest that it can interact with the transforming proteins of different DNA tumour viruses. In addition, it has been established that mutations in the Rb gene are also present in a variety of other human tumours, including mammary and lung cancer.

Two other tumour suppressor genes which, however, behave as dominant mutations, are the earlier described *erbA* gene and the *p53* gene.

In general, the consistent occurrence of a specific chromosomal aberration in a certain type of cancer is an indication for the location of a tumour suppressor gene in this region. This can, similar to the case of retinoblastoma, be a tool for the isolation and subsequent characterisation of the specific gene involved.

Oncogenes in Model Systems of Human Prostatic Cancer

So far, our knowledge of genes involved in neoplastic growth of prostatic cells is very limited. This holds both for animal model systems and human prostatic cancer. At present there is no strong indication that a DNA or RNA tumour virus is involved in the aetiology of prostatic cancer. In addition, evidence that a specific chromosomal aberration is an early event in the development of prostatic cancer is not available. Direct analysis of the genomic DNA of prostate tumour cell lines revealed in only one case (the human PC3 tumour cell line) the presence of an amplified oncogene (*c-myc*) [10,11]. However, not all PC3 sublines seem to contain amplified *c-myc* genes and *myc* amplification cannot be found in other prostate cancer cell lines or in primary tumours [10,12 and J.Trapman, unpublished results].

Another approach that has been undertaken is the analysis of cellular oncogene expression at the mRNA or protein level. In a series of 8 variant Dunning prostate carcinomas, expression of *myc*, *fos*, *p53*, *sis*, *neu*, *Ha-ras* and *Ki-ras* has been investigated and compared with the expression levels in the normal rat prostate [13,14]. In general, expression levels of the various oncogene mRNA's was higher in the tumour cell lines than in the normal prostate. However, no correlation with growth characteristics of the cells could be found. Similarly, analysis of proto-oncogene mRNA expression (including *ras*) in different human prostate tumour cell lines revealed no strong correlation with growth properties, although also in this study a high expression level of *c-myc* mRNA was observed [15]. In contrast, data obtained by Fan suggest that there is a relationship between the level of p21 *ras* protein expression and the metastatic capacity of subpopulations of the LRVA-4 prostate tumour cell line [16].

The *v-Ha-ras* gene has been introduced in a low-metastatic variant Dunning tumour cell line by gene transfer techniques [17]. Due to the expression of the *v-Ha-ras* gene, this cell line was converted into high-metastatic cells. Elegant gene transfer studies have recently been reported by Thompson et al. [18]. Recombinant nonreplicating retroviruses containing the *v-Ha-ras* and/or the *v-myc* gene were constructed and used for *in vitro* infection of the fetal mouse urogenital sinus, which can differentiate into prostate tissue. Subsequently, the organ reconstitutions were grafted under the renal capsule of male hosts. After several weeks, morphogenesis and functional differentiation of the transplant were investigated. Only the viruses containing both the *ras* and *myc* gene induced rapidly proliferating primary carcinomas. However, additional genetic alterations were also detected in the tumour cells. These experiments are no proof for a role of *myc* and\or *ras* in "spontaneously" developing human prostatic carcinoma. In fact, the rapid proliferation of the tumour argues against such a role. On the other hand, the experiments nicely illustrate that more than one event is needed to obtain a malignant (prostate) tumour.

Oncogenes in Human Prostatic Cancer

The oncogenes that have been analysed most intensively in primary human prostate cancer are the *ras* genes. In 3T3 cell transformation experiments, using DNA from prostate tumours, the presence of an activated *Ki-ras* gene could be established in one out of 8 samples [12]. There are no data available on the incidence of mutations in the *ras* genes as determined by direct structural analysis of codon 12,13 and 61. However, because most prostate tumours are not very aggressive, it would be a surprise if a high incidence of *ras* mutations could be found.

Data about the expression levels of the *ras* proto-oncogenes are conflicting. Viola et al. [19] demonstrated in an immunohistochemical study an increased expression of the p21 *ras* protein in tumour cells compared with normal prostate epithelial cells. They also showed a strong correlation between the p21 expression level and the tumour grade. However, in a more recent study by Varma et al., these results could not be confirmed [20]. Analysis of *Ha-ras* and *Ki-ras* mRNA expression indicates a small increase in high-grade prostate carcinomas [21].

Reports on properties and expression levels of other oncogenes are limited and fragmentary. Similar to the results found in prostate cell lines, expression of *myc* mRNA seems enhanced in prostate tumours, *sis* mRNA levels are increased in high-grade carcinomas; *fos* mRNA levels are low in undifferentiated tumours. In addition, the number of EGF receptors is increased in prostate tumour preparations [21,22]. A major problem in this type of experiments is the heterogeneity of the samples analysed. Another drawback, as also pointed out by the authors, is the lack of an appropriate control. Therefore, the results obtained so far, although of importance, have to be considered with great caution.

The Androgen Receptor

The development and the function of the prostate gland are androgen dependent. Similarly, the growth of the majority of prostate tumours depends on androgens. Depletion of testosterone and blockade of androgen action are important therapeutic interventions. Ultimately, however, androgen-independent tumours continue to proliferate. Possible mechanisms of androgen-independent growth are: 1. Bypass of the androgen-dependent process by an alternative (tumour specific) route. 2. Modification of the androgen-dependent pathway during therapy. 3. Outgrowth of an androgen-independent subpopulation of cells, which was already present before the therapy started. To understand the mechanism of androgen-depen-

dent and androgen-independent cell growth, knowledge of the molecular mechanism of androgen action is of major importance. This knowledge can also be applied for improvement of diagnosis and therapy of prostate cancer.
Androgens exert their function by interacting with the intracellular androgen receptor. The androgen-receptor complex is able to regulate transcription of specific target genes. Recently, the structure of the androgen receptor has been elucidated [23-26]. It is a member of a large family of structurally related ligand-dependent transcription modifiers [27,28]. Other members of this family include receptors for other steroid hormones, the vitamin D3 receptor and receptors for thyroid hormones and retinoic acid. They all show a similar structure with 3 different functional domains. The C-terminal part of the protein is essential for ligand binding; the DNA-binding domain is composed of two so-called "zinc finger" motifs and is highly conserved; the N-terminal domain is variable and plays a role in modulation of gene expression.
The molecular cloning of androgen receptor cDNA provides the opportunity to synthesise large amounts of the purified receptor. In addition, specific mutations can be introduced in the molecule. These methods can now be applied for detailed structure/function analysis of the steroid binding domain of the receptor. The outcome of these studies will be of great importance for the development of new antiandrogens.
cDNA probes and specific antibodies, which have been developed recently [25,29,30], can be applied for the study of androgen receptor structure and expression in androgen-dependent and androgen-independent prostate tumours.

Conclusions and Future Prospects

Although the knowledge of the molecular biology of cancer has increased enormously during the last decade, it is far from complete. Especially in the case of human cancer many problems still have to be resolved.
The molecular biology of prostate cancer is poorly documented. The main reasons for this are the lack of sufficient animal and *in vitro* models, the low growth rate of the tumour and its heterogeneity. In addition, no simple tools (viral aetiology, specific chromosome translocations, gene amplifications) are as yet available to tackle the problem. Hopefully, studies of prostate cell biology including prostate differentiation and development will lead to increasing knowledge on regulatory processes in the normal prostate, which can be compared with the properties of prostate tumours. Although much remains to be learned, tools are available to investigate one aspect of the prostate: the function of the androgen receptor in androgen-dependent and androgen-independent prostate tumour growth. Whether this will lead to improvement of diagnosis and therapy is still an unresolved question.

REFERENCES

1 Weinberg RA: The action of oncogenes in the cytoplasm and nucleus. Science 1985 (230):770-776
2 Bishop JM: The molecular genetics of cancer. Science 1987 (235):305-311
3 Watson JD, Hopkins NH, Roberts JW, Steitz JA and Weiner AM. In: Molecular Biology of the Gene. The Benjamin/Cummings Publishing Company, Menlo Park, Cal. 1987 pp 962-1096
4 Weinberg RA: Finding the anti-oncogene. Scient Amer 1988 (Sept):44-51
5 Weinberg RA: Positive and negative controls on cell growth. Biochemistry 1989 (28):8263-8269
6 Sager R: Tumor suppressor genes: the puzzle and the promise. Science 1989 (246):1406-1412
7 Bos JL: Ras oncogenes in human cancer: a review. Cancer Res 1989 (49):4682-4689
8 Damm K, Thompson CC and Evans RM: Protein encoded by v-erbA functions as a thyroid-hormone receptor antagonist. Nature 1989 (339):593-597
9 Sap J, Munoz A, Schmitt J, Stunnenberg H and Vennström B: Repression of transcription mediated at a thyroid hormone element by the v-erb-A oncogene product. Nature 1989 (340):242-244
10 Trapman J, Jenster G, Riegman P, Klaassen P, Van der Korput JAGM, Van Steenbrugge GJ and Romijn JC: Expression of (proto)oncogenes and genes encoding growth factors, growth factor receptors and prostate antigen in human prostate carcinoma cell lines. Progr Cancer Res Ther 1988 (35):102-109
11 Fukumoto M, Shevrin DH and Roninson IB: Analysis of gene amplification in human tumor cell lines. Proc Natl Acad Sci USA 1988 (85):6846-6850
12 Peehl DM, Wehner N and Stamey TA: Activated Ki-ras oncogene in human prostatic carcinoma. The Prostate 1987 (10):281-289
13 Cooke DB, Quarmby VE, Mickey DD, Isaacs JT and French FS: Oncogene expression in prostate cancer: Dunning R3327 rat dorsal prostatic adenocarcinoma system. The Prostate 1988 (13):263-272
14 Cooke DB, Quarmby VE, Petrusz P, Mickey DD, Der CJ, Isaacs JT and French FS: Expression of ras proto-oncogenes in the Dunning R3327 rat prostatic adenocarcinoma system. The Prostate 1988 (13):273-287
15 Rijnders AWM, Van der Korput JAGM, Van Steenbrugge GJ, Romijn JC and Trapman J: Expression of cellular oncogenes in human prostatic carcinoma cell lines. Biochem Biophys Res Commun 1985 (132):548-554
16 Fan K: Heterogeneous subpopulations of human prostatic adenocarcinoma cells: potential usefulness of p21 protein as a predictor for bone metastasis. J Urol 1988 (139):318-322
17 Treiger B and Isaacs J: Expression of a transfected v-harvey- ras oncogene in a Dunning rat prostate adenocarcinoma and the development of high metastatic ability. J Urol 1988 (140):1580-1586
18 Thompson TC, Southgate J, Kitchener G and Land H: Multistage carcinogenesis induced by ras and myc oncogenes in a reconstituted organ. Cell 1989 (56):917-930
19 Viola MV, Fronowitz F, Oravez S, Deb S, Finkel G, Lundy J, Hand P, Thor A and Schlom J: Expression of ras oncogene p21 in prostate cancer. N Engl J Med 1986 (314):133-137
20 Varma VA, Austin GE and O'Connell AC: Antibodies to ras oncogene p21 proteins lack immunohistochemical specificity for neoplastic epithelium in human prostate tissue. Arch Pathol Lab Med 1989 (113):16-19
21 Phillips MEA, Ferro MA, Smith PJB and Davies P: Intranuclear androgen receptor deployment and protooncogene expression in human diseased prostate: Urol Int 1987 (42):115-119
22 Davies P, Eaton CL, France TD and Philips MEA: Growth factor receptors and oncogene expression in prostate cells: Am J Clin Oncol 1988 (11):S1-S7
23 Trapman J, Klaassen P, Kuiper GGJM, Van der Korput JAGM, Faber PW, Van Rooij HCJ, Geurts van Kessel A, Voorhorst MM, Mulder E and Brinkmann AO: Cloning, structure and expression of cDNA encoding the human androgen receptor. Biochem Biophys Res Commun 1988 (153):241-248
24 Chang C, Kokontis J and Liao S: Structural analysis of complementary DNA and amino acid sequences of human and rat androgen receptors. Proc Natl Acad Sci USA 1988 (85):7211-7215
25 Lubahn DB, Joseph DR, Sar M, Tan J, Higgs HN, Larson RE, French FS and Wilson EM: The human androgen receptor: complementary deoxyribonucleic acid cloning, sequence analysis and gene expression in prostate. Mol Endocrinol 1988 (2):1265- 1275
26 Faber PW, Kuiper GGJM, Van Rooij HCJ, Van der Korput JAGM, Brinkmann AO and Trapman J: The N-terminal domain of the human androgen receptor is encoded by one, large exon. Mol Cell Endocrinol 1989 (61):257-262
27 Green S and Chambon P: Nuclear receptors enhance our understanding of transcription regulation. Trends Genet 1988 (4):309-314
28 Evans RM: The steroid and thyroid hormone receptor superfamily. Science 1988 (240):889-895

29 Chang C, Whelan CT, Popovich TC, Kokontis J and Liao S: Fusion proteins containing androgen receptor sequences and their use in the production of poly- and monoclonal anti-androgen receptor antibodies. Endocrinol 1989 (123):1097-1099

30 Van Laar JH, Voorhorst-Ogink MM, Zegers N, Boersma W, Claassen E, Van der Korput JAGM, Ruizeveld de Winter JA, Van der Kwast TH, Mulder E, Trapman J and Brinkmann AO: Characterization of antibodies against the N-terminal domain of the human androgen receptor. Mol Cell Endocrinol 1989 (67):29-38

The Endocrinological Basis for Hormonal Therapy of Prostate Tumours

M. Motta

Department of Endocrinology, University of Milano, Via Balzaretti 9, 20133 Milano, Italy

The growth and the activity of the normal prostate is largely dependent upon androgens, a characteristic that is frequently retained (80% of all cases of prostatic cancer) by the prostatic cells which develop into neoplastic cells (either benign: benign prostatic hypertrophy, BPH, or malignant: prostatic carcinoma). This concept is supported by the fact that the lack of testicular function (either due to castration or to hypopituitarism prior to the age of 40) prevents the occurrence of prostatic tumours in males over 55 years of age. It has been reported that the members of a Russian sect who undergo ritual castration before the age of 35 never exhibit the symptoms of BPH and have a prostate smaller than normal (see [1] for review).

Since the fundamental observation of Huggins and his colleagues [2] who established the hormone dependence of prostatic cancers, the treatment of these diseases has been aimed essentially either at inhibiting androgen secretion or at interfering with their action at the prostatic level. Endocrine therapy of prostatic carcinoma includes orchidectomy, hypophysectomy, adrenalectomy, administration of oestrogens and progestagens, treatment with androgen antagonists (antiandrogens or inhibitors of androgen biosynthesis and metabolism) and, more recently, administration of potent, long-acting agonistic analogues of LHRH, either alone or in combination with antiandrogens.

A better understanding of the mechanisms by which each of the endocrine treatments exhibits its antitestosterone effects, is of fundamental importance for an optimal clinical utilisation of the drugs.

This chapter will first summarise the roles played by the different hormones involved in the regulation of the function of the prostate. Subsequently, the mode of action on which the different endocrine treatments are based will be presented. Attention will be paid not only to the therapeutical approaches that have already been tested with promising results in clinical trials, but also to the more recent ones, which are expected to be of clinical significance.

It is not the aim of this chapter to discuss the choice of the most effective, safe and least troublesome method among the various endocrine regimens available, or to indicate which patients would benefit from endocrine treatments. These two points will be dealt with in other chapters in this volume.

Endocrine Regulation and Physiology of the Prostate

Androgens

Androgens play a key role in the complex process of controlling prostatic function and growth (Figs. 1 and 3). The primary source of androgens resides in the testes, but a small contribution comes also from the adrenals. The testes secrete about 5 to 10 mg of testosterone a day and also contribute approximately 30% of the plasma androstenedione, either by direct secretion or by peripheral conversion of testosterone [3]. In plasma, testosterone is reversibly bound to the sex hormone-binding globulin (SHBG), so that only about 2% of total plasma testos-

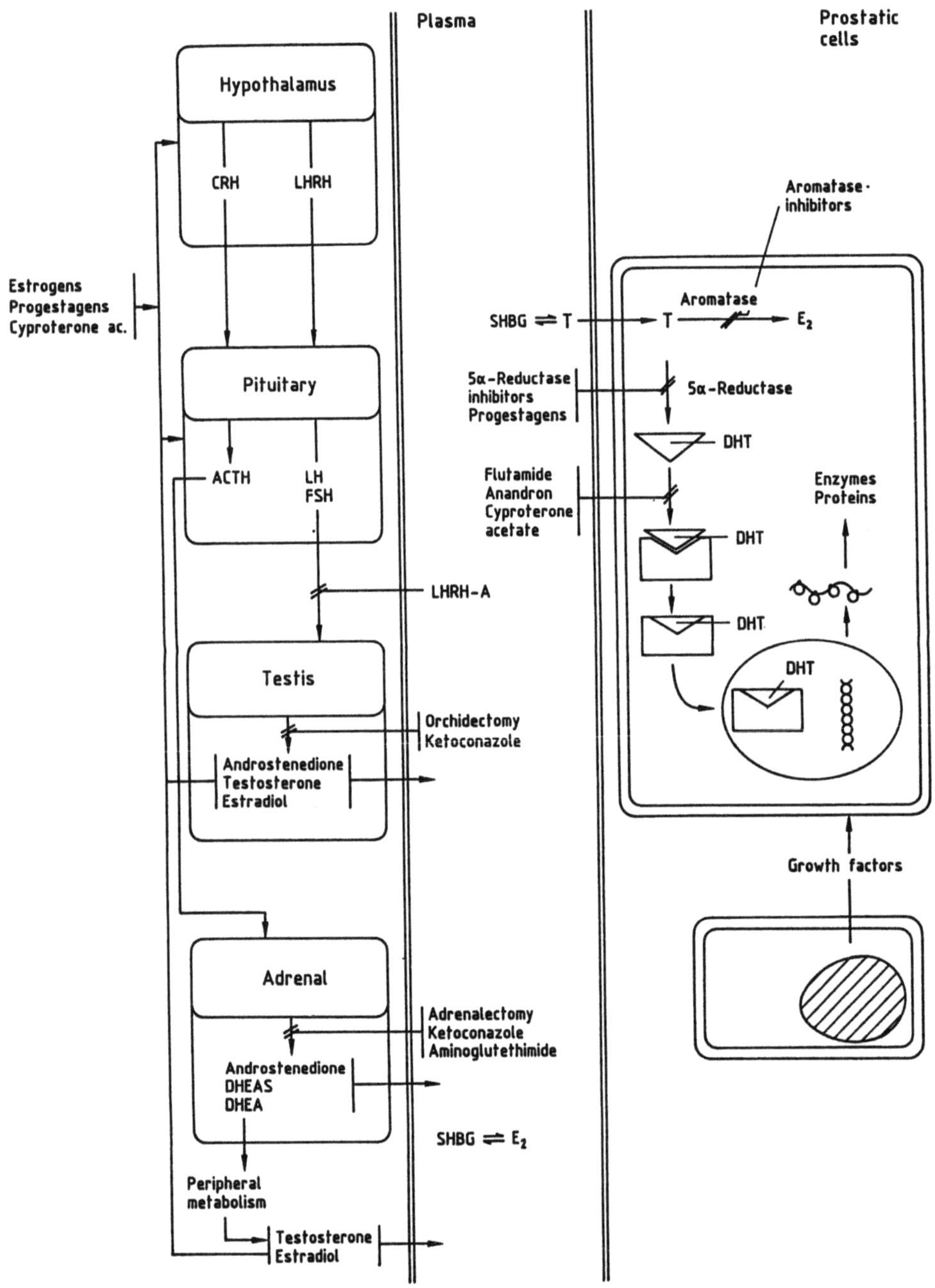

Fig. 1. Schematic representation of the endocrine control of the function of the prostate

terone remains in a free unbound state; it is this free fraction which is considered to be the biologically active form of the hormone [3].

Androgens of testicular origin (in particular testosterone) are synthesised and released by the Leydig cells in response to stimulation by luteinising hormone (LH). This pituitary hormone is, in turn, controlled by the hypothalamic LH releasing hormone (LHRH), which is secreted into the hypophysial portal circulation and reaches the anterior pituitary. To promote the release of the gonadotrophins (LH and follicle stimulating hormone or FSH), LHRH binds to specific receptors localised on the membrane of the gonadotropic cells. Plasma levels of testosterone, in turn, regulate the release of both LHRH and gonadotrophins by a negative feedback mechanism, thought to operate both at the hypothalamic and the pituitary level [4].

The main androgens of adrenal origin (which account for about 10% of the total amount of circulating androgens) are dehydroepiandrosterone (DHEA), its sulphate (DHEAS) and androstenedione. These steroids undergo metabolic conversion to testosterone and dihydrotestosterone (DHT), either in plasma or in the prostate itself (see below); data are available which indicate that the human prostatic tissue has the ability to take up and metabolise adrenal androgens [5]. The adrenal production of androgens is controlled by the adrenocorticotropic hormone (ACTH), which is under the influence of the hypothalamic corticotrophin releasing hormone (CRH).

Recently, adrenal androgens have been assigned a role in promoting tumour growth [6,7]. The concept that the adrenals may influence prostatic growth and function received support from the work of Tullner [8], who found that the administration of ACTH to immature castrated rats promoted the growth of the ventral prostate, while there was no response in adrenalectomised animals. However, a recent study by Walsh's group [9] indicates that, in patients with hypogonadotropic hypogonadism but with normal adrenal glands, the prostates at autopsy are very small and atrophic. These contradictory findings suggest that it is still a matter of debate whether adrenal androgens are as important as those of testicular origin in favouring the growth of prostatic tumours.

In the prostate, testosterone does not act as such, but serves as a prohormone for the formation of different 5alpha-reduced metabolites that mediate the majority of the intracellular processes under androgenic control. A large group of *in vitro* and *in vivo* studies has unequivocally established that the prostate, as other androgen-sensitive peripheral structures (seminal vesicles, sebaceous glands, etc.), metabolises testosterone into 5alpha-androstane-17beta-ol-3-one (DHT), 5alpha-androstane-3alpha, 17beta-diol (3alpha-diol), and 5alpha-androstane-3beta, 17beta-diol (3beta-diol) [10-12]. These conversions occur under the influence of an enzymatic complex which includes a 5alpha-reductase and two 3alpha- and 3beta-hydroxysteroid dehydrogenases. In the prostate, testosterone is also converted to androstenedione, 5alpha-androstanedione and androsterone (see Fig. 2). These metabolic processes have been studied extensively in animal models. It is likely that testosterone is metabolised in a similar manner by the normal human prostatic tissue; however, the difficulty in obtaining normal human material for these types of studies is self-evident.

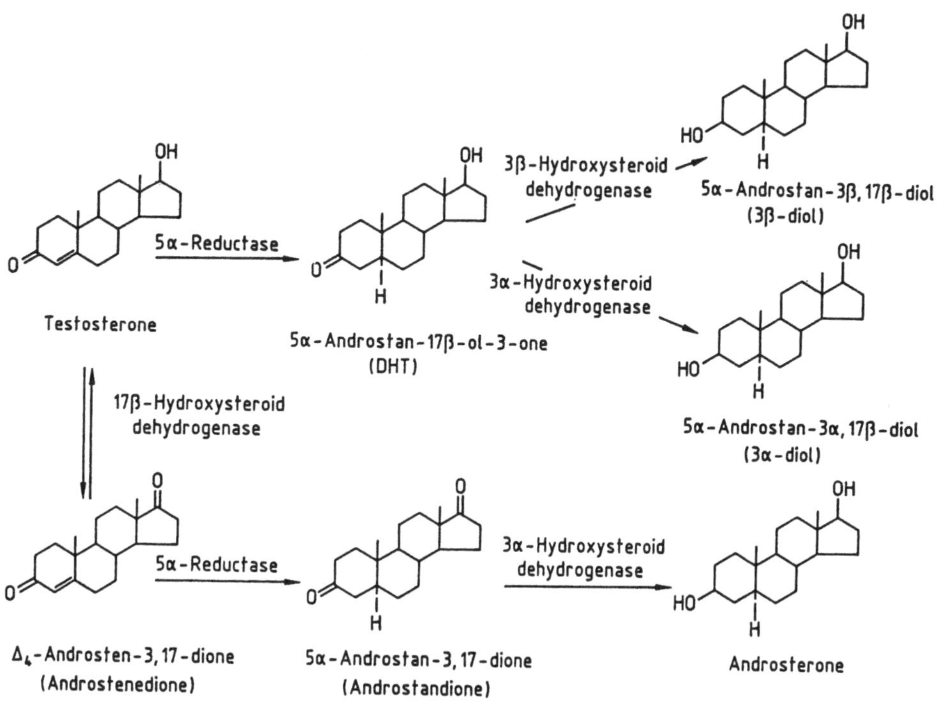

Fig. 2. Schematic representation of the metabolism of testosterone

Studies on the mechanism of action of androgens in the prostate demonstrate the important role of the conversion of testosterone to DHT, and indicate this hormone as the active intracellular androgen upon which the growth and the function of the prostate depend [13,14]. To exert its influence on cell function, DHT has to be bound to specific androgenic receptors. These receptors, which have been shown to be present in the normal prostate [15,16], bind testosterone also, but with a lower affinity (4 to 5 times). Consequently, DHT represents 90% or more of the steroids bound by the receptors present in the prostate. According to recent evidence, these receptors are predominantly present in the cell nuclei. Following binding of DHT to its receptor, the receptor undergoes a process of activation which allows the binding of the receptor-hormone complex to an acceptor site located on the chromatin; this directs the transcription of stored genetic material by increasing synthesis of specific messenger RNAs, which, in turn, lead to protein synthesis and to the specific response of the cell (growth, secretion, etc.).

The prominent role of DHT in the control of prostatic growth is underlined by the following evidence: a) in males with the 5alpha-reductase deficiency syndrome, the prostate is considerably decreased in size or completely absent; b) similarly, the prostate does not develop in patients affected by the testicular feminisation syndrome, who have a deficiency of androgen receptors despite their male genotype; c) DHT is more active than other androgens in stimulating cell hyperplasia of prostatic tissue in several experimental models *in vivo* and *in vitro* (see [1] for references).

DHT represents also the predominant steroid hormone in the diseased prostate; BPH is frequently associated with high tissue accumulation of DHT and increased tissue 5alpha-reductase activity [17,18]. By contrast, in malignant tissue, the 5alpha-reductase activity and the formation of DHT seem to be diminished; this decrease seems to be related to the histological differentiation of the tumour. In prostatic cancer, the testosterone metabolism appears mainly to follow the oxidative pathway with the formation of androstenedione [19] (see Fig. 2). Moreover, androgen receptors are also present in the pathological prostate and retain the characteristics of those present in normal cells [20].

Oestrogens

Other steroid hormones too, such as oestrogens, seem to be involved in the control of prostatic function. Oestrogens, which originate from the aromatisation of androgens, are produced in small amounts by testicular tissue; in males, the majority of circulating oestrogens derive from the peripheral aromatisation of precursors of adrenal (androstenedione) and testicular (testoster-one and androstenedione) origin. Similarly to testosterone, oestradiol is bound to SHBG and, through a negative feedback mechanism, influences the release of both LHRH and gonadotrophins [4] (see Fig. 1).

Although the exact role of oestrogens in the prostate has not been fully established, oestrogens have been shown to stimulate, either by themselves or in synergism with androgens, prostatic growth and secretion [21,22]. These observations, together with the finding that oestrogen receptors are present in the prostate [16,20], seem to suggest that these hormones act directly upon the gland.

Increasing evidence indicates that oestrogens may also participate in the development of BPH [18,23]; it has been reported that the tissue concentrations of oestrogens and oestrogen receptors are higher in the malignant gland than in BPH [24]. Support for the possible involvement of oestrogens in the pathogenesis of prostatic diseases comes from recent studies of Stone et al. [25] and Kaburagi et al. [26], who have found that the prostate has the capacity for aromatising androgens to oestrogens. Whether the *in situ* formation of oestrogens is more relevant than oestrogens derived peripherally from the precursors for the induction of BPH still remains to be established.

Peptide Hormones

The growth of the prostate can also be influenced by peptide hormones. Those which have been studied most extensively are prolactin and growth hormone (GH) and, more

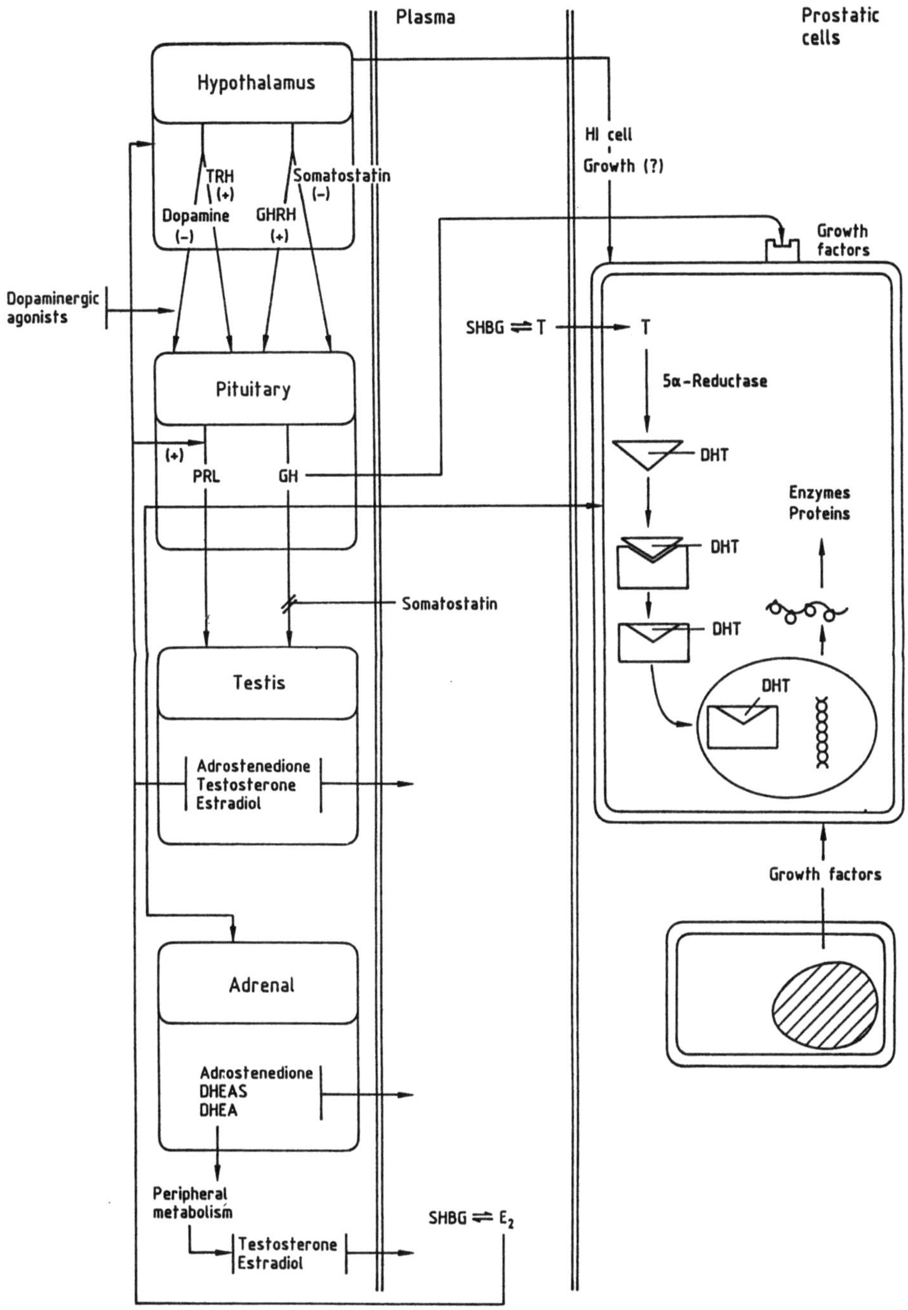

Fig. 3. Schematic representation of the endocrine control of the function of the prostate

recently, the tissue growth factors have also received some attention.

Prolactin

The secretion of prolactin is mainly regulated by an inhibitory influence from the hypothalamus; the prolactin inhibiting factor is identified with dopamine; once this principle is released into the hypophysial portal vessels, it inhibits the secretion of prolactin [27]. Conversely, oestrogens and TRH (thyrotrophin releasing hormone) stimulate prolactin secretion; oestrogens appear to act via central nervous regulatory centres [27] (Fig. 3). Hyperprolactinaemia is frequently observed in prostatic cancer patients undergoing oestrogen treatment [28].

Prolactin exerts its effects a) on the testes, where it acts synergistically with LH to stimulate testosterone secretion [29]; b) on the adrenals, where it promotes the release of

DHEA, DHEAS and androstenedione [30]; and c) via a recently suggested direct mitogenic action on prostatic cells [31], where receptors for this pituitary hormone have been localised [32]. As a consequence, prolactin may promote the growth of the prostate independently of androgens. Prolactin may also enhance the responses of the prostate to androgens, by acting synergistically with testosterone in promoting the growth of the gland, and by influencing the uptake of testosterone and the intraprostatic metabolism of androgens [32,33]. On the basis of these observations, it is currently believed that prolactin plays a regulatory role in the growth, maintenance and function of the prostate.
Prolactin seems to exert similar effects also on the diseased human prostate. A higher and faster uptake of testosterone has been observed in BPH patients whose plasma prolactin levels were stimulated with chlorpromazine than in untreated subjects [34]. However, because of the complexity of its actions, the involvement of prolactin in the development and maintenance of prostatic cancer is far from being completely understood.

GH

The secretion of GH is regulated by 2 hypothalamic hormones, a stimulating one, GHRH (growth hormone releasing hormone) and an inhibiting one, GHIH (growth hormone release inhibiting hormone, somatostatin) (Fig. 3). The growth promoting action of GH is mediated by the somatomedins, a group of structurally related polypeptides (see below), which seem to exert a negative feedback on GH release by stimulating somatostatin secretion, and by a direct effect on the pituitary where they block the action of GHRH [35]. Since GH appears to be the major regulator of plasma somatomedin levels, it might be expected that the effects of GH on the prostate are mediated by the somatomedins.
The possible participation of GH in the control of prostatic growth is still insufficiently understood. However, the observations that the administration of GH and ACTH to hypophysectomised castrated rats stimulates prostatic growth [36], and that GH levels are higher in patients with metastatic prostatic cancer than in patients without metastases [37], indicate that this hormone plays a role in the progression of the tumour. This is supported by recent findings showing that GH is localised in human prostatic tumours [38], and that this tissue possesses specific binding sites for GH [38].

Tissue growth factors

Tissue growth factors, which include many peptides (epidermal growth factor, EGF; transforming growth factor, TGF-alpha and beta; fibroblast growth factor, FGF; nerve growth factor, NGF; IGFI or somatomedin C, etc.), form a class of regulatory molecules with potent mitogenic activity. They exert their effects by binding to specific receptors present on the cell surface and by acting mainly through a paracrine mode of action (see [39] for review). Additionally, since these factors have biological effects on the same cell where they are produced and where their receptors are present, they are able to stimulate cellular growth also in an autocrine fashion [40]. While most of the growth factors studied exhibit growth promoting activities, TGF-beta has the peculiarity of showing dual effects, causing either stimulation or inhibition of cell growth [41,42]. These effects seem to be influenced by other growth factors [42]. For example, it has been found that, in the presence of EGF, TGF-beta displays inhibitory activity, yet in the presence of PDGF, TGF-beta is stimulatory; this indicates that TGF-beta acts either synergistically or antagonistically with other growth factors. This observation suggests then that, in order to ascertain a specific role for the growth factors on the mechanism of abnormal prostatic growth, the activity of each growth factor should be analysed individually.
Recent studies have suggested that the growth of the prostate can be altered by a number of different proteinaceous growth factors deriving either from the prostate itself or from other tissues (see [39] for review). A number of mitogenic activities have been described in the human prostate and, in some cases, their identity with known growth factors has been proven [43-46]. Nishi et al. [46] reported partial purification of a prostatic growth factor, related to the epidermal growth factor. Mydlo and colleagues [47] have isolated a

growth factor from human prostatic tissue which belongs to the family of basic FGF. Crabb et al. [48] have found a substance called "prostatrophin" deriving from the bovine brain which is mitogenic for human prostatic cells. This polypeptide is homologous to acidic FGF. The prostate contains, in addition to the growth factors, also the receptors to which the mitogens bind. Receptors for EGF (which also bind TGF-alpha) [49] and for TGF-beta have been demonstrated in the human prostate, while the characterisation of the receptor for FGF is still incompletely defined.

The diseased prostate also contains high concentrations of growth factors [50,51] (see [39] for references) and of their specific receptors [49,52]. Their presence in both prostatic cancer and BPH may suggest a role for these factors in the pathogenesis of these diseases, and may represent an important mechanism of growth control. It is also possible that qualitative as well as quantitative differences in the growth factors present in the gland might be responsible for the differential pathogenesis of BPH and prostatic cancer. Nishi et al. [53] have measured the content of several growth factors in tissue extracts of normal and pathological human prostates (BPH and prostatic cancer). They found that BPH tissue contains the largest amount of growth factors among the 3 groups of prostate considered. Tumour tissue seems to contain half the concentration of growth factors present in BPH. Normal prostates have a very low concentration of these peptides. However, independently of the amount of growth factors present in the prostate, it seems that normal and cancer cells respond to the different growth factors in a similar way [54]. The importance of growth factors and of their receptors in cancer is stressed by the finding that oncogenes might, in fact, be the genes coding for growth factors and their receptors.

In the light of these considerations, it might be discussed whether androgens, although important for the development, differentiation and maintenance of the prostate, represent just a single predominant component of a complex of regulatory mechanisms, in which a role is also played by the growth factors. Support for this hypothesis comes from the observation that androgens do not seem to exert a direct mitogenic action in isolated epithelial cells [55,56]; consequently, it might be suggested that, also *in vivo*, the mitogenic effect of androgens might not be direct, but rather mediated through the modulation of the effects of one or more of the growth factors. It has been shown [57] that androgen removal results in increased binding of EGF to its receptors, while androgen replacement causes a decrease in the number of EGF receptors (i.e., androgens down-regulate EGF receptors) [57]. It may then be postulated that androgen deprivation may induce growth factor receptors which, in turn, may promote cell growth and prevent the complete regression of the prostate; this mechanism may maintain the pool of reserve cells from which the prostate may regenerate following androgen treatment. If the interaction of androgens with other growth regulating factors is critical to prostatic growth, one might be tempted to suggest that prostatic cancer is the result of an imbalance between androgens and growth factors.

From these preliminary observations it emerges that it has still to be clearly defined a) whether there is *in situ* production of the growth factors in the prostate, b) how these factors interact with other systems of hormonal control of prostatic growth, and c) how they are involved in the malignant transformation of prostatic cells. Further studies are obviously needed before new types of treatment of prostatic tumours are developed.

Mechanism of Action of the Different Therapeutical Approaches

The endocrine control of the growth and function of the normal prostate is a complex process, the crucial event of which is to maintain an adequate supply of androgens, in particular testosterone, to the gland. It is not yet totally clear how many of the factors involved in such a regulation (see above) are equally responsible for the growth and evolution of prostatic tumours. At any rate, the dependence upon testosterone of many of the prostatic tumours is undoubted. Therefore, the rationale of any endocrine treatment of these diseases is, for the time being, either to lower testosterone levels in the general circulation or to interfere with the metabolism and the biological effects of the hormone at the cellular level. As will be shown below, the mode of action of each hormonal manipulation is quite different, since they operate at different levels of the endocrine regulation of prostatic function.

Bilateral Orchidectomy

The most conventional and direct method for lowering plasma androgen levels to a minimum is to remove the primary source of testosterone by bilateral orchidectomy. After removal of the testes, it can be predicted that any residual testosterone in the circulation is of adrenal origin. Secondary endocrine effects occur after orchidectomy: as expected, these involve mainly the hypothalamo-pituitary axis with a permanent increase of plasma levels of LH and FSH, as a consequence of the loss of the negative feedback effect exerted by testosterone on LHRH and gonadotrophin secretion (see Fig. 1).

Oestrogens

Drugs with oestrogenic properties are thought to act primarily by inhibiting the activity of the hypothalamo-pituitary system through a negative feedback mechanism (see Fig. 1). This effect leads to a fall in the secretion of LH, which results in the decrease of testosterone synthesis by testicular tissue [4].

It must be pointed out that oestrogenic compounds may also decrease the synthesis of testosterone acting directly at the testicular level, and exert a direct local action on the prostate, as indicated by a decrease in the intraprostatic conversion of testosterone to DHT by inhibition of DNA synthesis, etc. [58-60]. However, it should be emphasised once again that oestrogenic drugs develop their antitumoural action mainly because of their feedback effect on the hypothalamo-pituitary axis. All the other effects occur when oestrogens are given in doses far exceeding the levels that can be achieved in patients without any marked side effects.

As mentioned previously, oestrogenic compounds increase plasma prolactin levels. This secondary effect could be relevant in the treatment of patients with prostatic cancer, since prolactin is able to influence the growth of the prostate, as reported in the preceding section. However, on the basis of the available clinical studies, it is unlikely that the doses of oestrogens used can induce an increase in plasma prolactin levels capable of affecting adrenal and/or testicular synthesis of androgens.

Oestrogenic drugs utilised to treat prostatic cancers are either non-steroidal synthetic compounds (such as diethylstilboestrol, diethylstilboestrol diphosphate, chlorotrianisene and dienoestrol) or steroids (such as polyoestradiol phosphate or oestradurin and ethinyloestradiol). It is obvious that the ideal agent of this type for the treatment of prostatic cancer should have a predominant antigonadotropic activity and a local antiandrogenic effect on prostatic tissue, but minimal oestrogenic side effects (gynaecomastia, effects on blood coagulation, etc.).

Progestagens

Progestational drugs, the most studied of which are megoestrol acetate and medrogestone [18,61], exert their effects directly on the hypothalamo-pituitary axis (see Fig. 1); by way of a negative feedback mechanism they inhibit LH release, thereby decreasing testicular secretion of testosterone [18]. Similarly to progesterone, they also prevent the transformation of testosterone to DHT, possibly by acting as preferential substrates for 5alpha-reductase; a decrease in the intraprostatic concentrations of DHT and a blockade of 5alpha-reductase activity are thus achieved [18,61-63]. Unlike oestrogens, progestagens do not increase serum levels of prolactin.

Androgen Antagonists

A more modern method of depriving prostatic cancer tissue of its major trophic stimulus, testosterone, is based on the utilisation of androgen antagonists. This class of substances includes both the antiandrogens and the inhibitors of androgen biosynthesis and metabolism.

Antiandrogens

Antiandrogens (such as cyproterone acetate, flutamide, anandron, etc.) are compounds that block the biological effects of testosterone within the target organ cell, by inhibiting the binding of DHT and testosterone to the androgenic receptors [64]. The antiandrogen-receptor complex does not bind to the chromatin, and, consequently, the hormonal effect on protein synthesis is prevented (see Fig. 1). Because of their mechanism of action, the antiandrogens are able to counteract the effect of androgens of both testicular and adrenal origin.

Despite the fact that antiandrogens have basically the same mechanism of action, their *in vivo* endocrine effects are quite different. A distinction is generally made between those substances which also have other endocrine properties (e.g., progestational and antigonadotropic activities) and the pure antiandrogens which have only antiandrogenic properties.

Cyproterone acetate belongs to the first category of antiandrogens. Since this compound possesses a strong progestational effect, it induces a reduction of plasma LH and FSH levels by activating the negative feedback mechanism at the hypothalamo-pituitary level, and consequently also inhibits the biosynthesis of testicular androgens [65]. At the same time, this steroid competes with androgens for the same receptors at the target cell level [65]. Thus, androgen deprivation in the case of cyproterone acetate is obtained in two ways: a) by inhibition of androgen biosynthesis through the suppression of gonadotrophin secretion, and b) by inhibition of the remaining (adrenal) androgens by an action at the receptorial level (see Fig. 1).

In contrast to cyproterone acetate, pure antiandrogens, such as flutamide and anandron, are devoid of progestational and antigonadotropic properties [66,67]. They only compete with androgens at their receptor sites, not only at the level of the prostate, but also of the hypothalamo-pituitary complex (where androgens exert their negative feedback effect) (see Fig. 1); as a result, LH secretion is increased and consequently, in the presence of the testes, the biosynthesis of testosterone is also increased [68]. However, due to the presence of the antiandrogen, the hormone cannot exert its action on the prostate.

Since these two classes of antiandrogens express their effects *in vivo* in a different way, this implies that they also have different clinical applications. Only antiandrogens of the cyproterone acetate type should be used as monotherapy in non-castrated patients, while both types of antiandrogens are useful when given in combination with castration (either surgical or medical). Cyproterone acetate seems to be more appropriate than pure antiandrogens in the initial phase of treatment with LHRH agonists, because it inhibits, at least partially, the oversecretion of testosterone (see below). Both types of antiandrogens should be equally qualified in combination with LHRH therapy, after down-regulation of the pituitary LHRH receptors has occurred (see below).

Recently, a new, potent, pure non-steroidal antiandrogen has been developed [69]. The peculiarity of this compound is represented by its selectivity of action for the peripheral androgen-dependent structures, when tested in various animal species [69]. Because of this property, it should have potential advantages over existing agents. Unlike cyproterone acetate, it does not have progestational properties. In contrast to flutamide and anandron, it produces negligible effects on serum LH and androgens, because the compound does not seem to cross the blood-brain barrier and, consequently, does not eliminate the negative feedback effect exerted by androgens. In addition, this molecule has a much longer half-life than flutamide; this would make this antiandrogen more suitable for medical use. Clinical trials are now in progress to validate the selectivity observed in rats and to assess the clinical benefit of the compound [70].

Inhibitors of androgen metabolism

So far, the approach of antagonising the effects of androgens has only been that of displacing androgens from their specific receptor sites. The demonstration that DHT and oestrogens are the mediators of trophic effects in the prostate, and that 5alpha-reductase and aromatase are the enzymes involved in the intracellular transformation of testosterone into DHT and oestrogens, respectively, may provide the basis for the development of new androgen antagonists which may offer additional opportunities for the treatment of prostatic diseases. It is obvious that, in the presence of these compounds, testosterone reaches its target structure, but is unable to exert its activity because of the absence of the intracellular transformation into DHT and/or oestrogens. 5Alpha-reductase inhibitors and aromatase inhibitors belong to this new class of androgen antagonists.

5Alpha-reductase inhibitors

Progesterone, megoestrol acetate and medrogesterone have all been reported to inhibit 5alpha-reductase [18,61,62]. However, these compounds possess other endocrine properties which prevail over that of inhibiting 5alpha-reductase activity.
Compounds whose primary mode of action is that of interfering with this enzyme have now been tested both *in vivo* and *in vitro* in different animal tissues [12,13,71,72]. It has been reported that, when given *in vivo*, they selectively inhibit testosterone-induced but not DHT-induced growth of the prostate of castrated rats [13] as well as of dogs [73]. However, most of these molecules have not yet been tested in clinical trials, because of the lack of adequate pharmacological and toxicological studies.
Only one compound of this series, MK-906 (N-2(-methyl-2-propyl)-3-oxo-4-aza-5alpha-androst-1-ene-17beta-carboxamide) is being extensively investigated in BPH subjects (see [1] for review). This drug is very potent and differs from all the 5alpha-reductase inhibitors mentioned so far in that it is effective at very low doses, and at these doses it blocks the formation of DHT locally in the prostate with minor effects (if any) on plasma testosterone levels [74]. Moreover, this compound is devoid of any toxic effect: no signs of renal, hepatic or other laboratory or clinical toxicity have been observed in patients treated with this drug [1].

Aromatase inhibitors

Aromatase inhibitors are those compounds that block the transformation of androgens to oestrogens, interfering with aromatase activity [75]. Since it has been suggested that oestrogens play a role in the development of prostatic tumours [18,23-25], it is conceivable that these compounds may prove to be useful in the treatment of these diseases. Particular attention has been paid to one of these molecules, namely 4-hydroxy-androstenedione; preliminary studies indicate that this compound is effective in prostatic diseases [75].
The approach of interfering with the metabolism of testosterone either with 5alpha-reductase inhibitors or with aromatase inhibitors yields definite advantages over the other types of treatment, because these new classes of drugs suppress the effect of testosterone at the target level, but leave the plasma concentrations of the hormone unmodified. Of course, much work has yet to be done, but the preliminary clinical results are highly promising and attractive.

LHRH Analogues

A radically different endocrine approach to reduce androgenic stimulation of prostatic cancer is the use of highly potent, long-acting LHRH analogues. These compounds became available soon after the structure of LHRH was elucidated [76]. Two different categories of LHRH analogues have been synthesised: a) the superactive agonists, in which the full pattern of activity of the original hormone is maintained, but which possess marked biological and pharmacological activities with a more prolonged duration of action, and b) the antagonistic analogues, which are devoid of intrinsic LHRH activity but are able to inhibit the activity of endogenous LHRH by interacting with its receptors at the pituitary level.

LHRH agonists

The most potent agonistic analogues of LHRH show the substitution of the amino acid in position 6 with a D amino acid (biodegradation is thus prevented), and the deletion of the amino acid in position 10 with the addition of an ethylamide group to the proline residue in position 9 (a higher affinity to receptors is thus achieved) [77].
The peculiarity of these analogues is that, depending on the doses and on the modality of administration, they are able both to stimu-

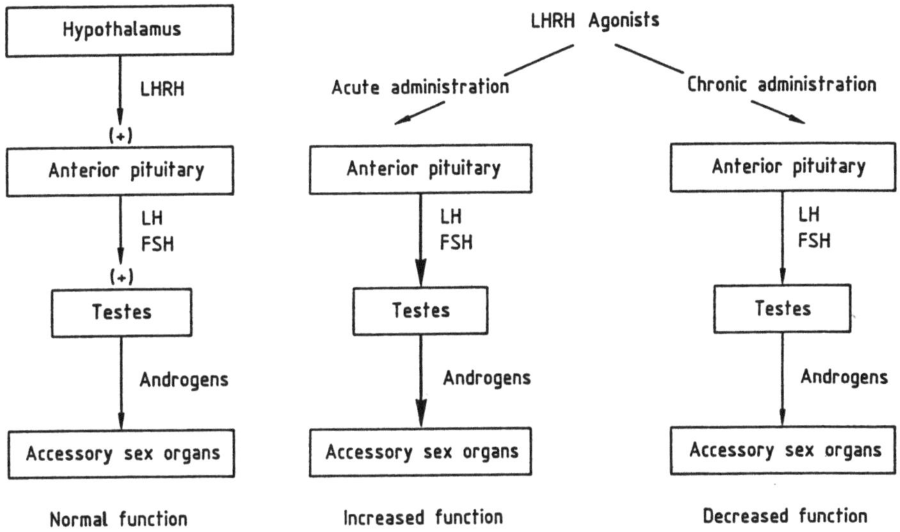

Fig. 4. Endocrine effect of acute and chronic administration of LHRH agonists

late and to inhibit gonadotrophin secretion. Acute and pulsatile administration of these analogues stimulates the secretion of gonadotrophins and results in increased testosterone production by the testes. By contrast, continuous administration of high doses of LHRH agonists causes an inhibition of LH and FSH release, and a subsequent suppression of testosterone secretion similar to that obtained by surgical castration [78] (Fig. 4). The so-called paradoxical effect (antigonadic) exhibited by LHRH agonists suggested the use of these compounds as antitumoural agents; this concept has been proven valid both in animal and in human studies [79].

Chronic administration of LHRH agonists can totally suppress gonadotrophin secretion by means of so-called down-regulation of the receptors for LHRH present at the pituitary level. As a result, the pituitary gland becomes refractory to further stimulation by endogenous LHRH and LHRH analogues; testicular androgen production is thus prevented [80]. However, it must be emphasised that all LHRH agonists, irrespective of their molecular structure or of the route of administration (subcutaneous, intramuscular, intranasal, etc.), induce, immediately following administration, an initial hypersecretion of gonadotrophins which is accompanied by an increase in testosterone release [78]. Only when LHRH-agonist plasma levels are sufficiently elevated, the pituitary receptors become blocked, down-regulation takes place and gonadal function is inhibited.

The pituitary gland does not seem to be the only target tissue for LHRH; extrapituitary effects have also been postulated. These include a) an action on the testes where LHRH agonists interfere with the biosynthesis of testosterone and down-regulate LHRH receptors [78]. However, this phenomenon has only been demonstrated in several animal species, but not in humans [78]; b) a direct action on the prostate itself. Specific binding sites for LHRH seem to be present in prostatic tumours [81]. Despite the multiple sites of action, the pituitary gland is believed to be the main target for LHRH agonists.

Treatment of prostatic tumours with LHRH agonists has two disadvantages: one is related to the initial LH-testosterone stimulatory period, during which there is an increase in the level of plasma prostatic acid phosphatase [82-84] and a consequent worsening of the disease-related symptoms; the second is due to the fact that LHRH therapy blocks only the secretion of testosterone deriving from the testes, but is ineffective on androgens of adrenal origin. This is why there are persisting, albeit low, levels of androgens in the circulation during LHRH-agonist treatment [7]. One way to overcome these disadvantages is to associate LHRH treatment with an antiandrogen, which prevents the binding of endogenous testosterone (either of testicular or adrenal origin) to its own receptors at the prostatic level (see sections on antiandrogens and adrenal suppression).

LHRH antagonists

LHRH-antagonistic analogues can be obtained either by removing the amino-acid residue in position 2, or by substituting it with a D amino acid, and by introducing a D amino acid in position 6 [77].
Similarly to LHRH agonists, LHRH antagonists induce an inhibition of gonadotrophin release and lower testosterone secretion, although their mechanism of action is totally different from that of the LHRH agonists [79]. These biologically inactive substances exert their effect at the receptorial level by preventing the binding of the endogenous LHRH to its pituitary receptors. Preliminary evidence suggests that these compounds are able to cause a significant reduction of prostatic tumour size and growth [85]. Suppression of Dunning rat prostate tumour growth has been obtained after chronic administration of LHRH antagonists [85]. In addition, the demonstration of the binding of one of the LHRH antagonists to plasma membrane obtained from the Dunning prostate tumour indicates that LHRH antagonists might also act directly on the prostate [86].
These preliminary experimental studies suggest that this class of compounds should also be considered for the treatment of prostatic carcinoma. Their use would avoid the transient stimulation of gonadotrophin and testosterone release that occurs initially in response to LHRH agonists, thus preventing a temporary flare-up of the disease [79]. However, LHRH antagonists have been tested in humans only in acute studies, and clinical data are not yet available on the effects of their chronic administration; a complete toxicological investigation is extremely necessary.
Since both LHRH agonists and antagonists have to be given by continuous administration, the development of long-acting pharmaceutical depot formulations seems to be an essential step towards their optimal clinical application [87].

Adrenal Suppression

Measurements of intraprostatic DHT concentrations have revealed unexpectedly elevated amounts of DHT in some prostatic cancers after orchidectomy, administration of oestrogens or of LHRH agonists, although these treatments cause a 90% decrease in serum testosterone levels [7,88]. This finding suggests that significant amounts of adrenal androgens may be converted to DHT within the tumour tissue after suppression of testicular androgenic production, and that the high tissue levels of DHT after surgical or medical castration seem to have a stimulatory effect on the development of prostatic cancers [7]. However, the lowest amount of androgens capable of stimulating prostatic tumour growth is not yet well defined [89]. Nevertheless, this possibility stresses the need to neutralise the action of androgens of adrenal origin and gives support to the concept of total androgen suppression for the treatment of prostatic cancer. Specific pharmacological treatments for removing adrenal androgens are available.

Aminoglutethimide

Aminoglutethimide produces a medical blockade of adrenocortical function by inhibiting the side-chain cleavage of cholesterol and subsequent hydroxylation, an early step in steroidogenesis. Consequently, the synthesis of androgens, cortisol and aldosterone is interrupted [90] (see Fig. 1). The deficiency of cortisol and aldosterone in the general circulation leads to hypersecretion of ACTH from the pituitary gland and justifies substitution therapy with hydrocortisone concomitantly with aminoglutethimide.

Ketoconazole

Ketoconazole is an orally administered synthetic imidazole derivative which is mostly used in the treatment of fungal diseases. High doses of this drug block the synthesis of testosterone in the testes and in the adrenal glands of animals and men [91] (see Fig. 1). Clinical studies with ketoconazole in prostatic cancers are scarce, and toxicity at the dose levels required is definitely incomplete.

Total androgen suppression

The availability of new drugs or combinations of drugs that are capable of suppressing the effect of both testicular and adrenal androgens has enabled the achievement of total androgen ablation in the treatment of prostatic cancers; in fact, the theory has been put forward that progression of tumour growth after conventional endocrine manipulation may result from the inadequate suppression of androgens of adrenal origin. This view is in contrast with the hypothesis that prostatic cancer is composed of both androgen-sensitive and androgen-insensitive cells, and that disease progression after hormonal therapy is largely the result of the proliferation of androgen-insensitive cells. However, total androgen suppression can be achieved theoretically by excluding all sources of androgen production or by blocking all androgen effects at the target cell level.

The most promising form of androgen ablation as first-line therapy for prostatic cancers appears to be the combination of an LHRH agonist with an antiandrogen [7].

In men with prostatic cancer, the combined administration of an LHRH analogue (either buserelin or leuprolide given as daily subcutaneous injection or as daily nasal spray) with an antiandrogen (either anandron or flutamide) prevents the rise in plasma prostatic acid phosphatase and prostate-specific antigen levels (two plasma markers of prostatic carcinoma, the latter of which is currently considered the best marker of prostatic carcinoma activity) [93], and has a beneficial effect on bone pain [94]. Furthermore, the levels of the markers decrease earlier and to a greater degree in men given combined therapy than in those treated only with the LHRH analogues [92]. The proportion of patients with complete or partial objective responses is higher (56%) than that achieved with an LHRH agonist alone (20-46%) [95]. Moreover, combination therapy appears to produce small but important improvements in both progression-free survival and overall survival (see [92,96] for references). From these studies it would emerge that combined therapy (LHRH agonist plus antiandrogen) is necessary not only during the first weeks of treatment to counteract the possible side effects of the initial transient increase in testosterone (flare-up), but also during chronic therapy to inhibit the action of the residual adrenal androgens [92,96]. However, the advantage of total androgen blockade obtained with combined therapy compared to that observed with LHRH-agonist monotherapy has not been confirmed by other clinical studies [97,98]. In addition, preliminary results obtained by an open, multicentre, randomised clinical study in which one group of patients was treated with a depot preparation of zoladex (an LHRH agonist) and the second group with the same agonist plus cyproterone acetate, does not seem to show any benefit for the combination over the agonist alone [99]. The debate is still open: the results obviously require confirmation from other larger studies using the same route of LHRH-agonist administration and longer periods of observation before drawing any final conclusions. For instance, it is possible that in the trials involving a long-lasting LHRH agonist, such as zoladex, the benefit of the combined therapy is not apparent; this may be related to improved compliance when the LHRH analogue is given as a monthly depot injection compared to a daily injection. Moreover, the better early objective response observed in patients treated with the combined therapy might become less apparent at longer times of observation (see [100] for review).

Somatostatin

Somatostatin, a 14 amino-acid containing cyclic peptide, was first isolated from the hypothalamus and subsequently found in the pancreatic islets and in the gut [101]. This hormone possesses multivalent actions: it inhibits hormone secretion (GH, insulin, glucagon and prolactin, etc.), DNA synthesis and cell proliferation [101].

Somatostatin in itself seems to be of limited value in the therapy of human disorders. The two major problems that limit the therapeutic effectiveness of somatostatin are its short half-life (i.e., its short duration of action after systemic administration due to its rapid disactivation by peptidases) and its marked diversity of action (i.e., its lack of selectivity for a given target cell or tissue).

Structural analogues of somatostatin have been synthesised in an effort to circumvent these problems [101]. Because somatostatin analogues possess the same properties as the native hormone, they could prove useful in treating certain forms of cancer as they might suppress the growth and/or secretory activity of the tumours [101].

Preliminary findings may suggest a possible application of these analogues in the management of prostatic cancer. Low doses of these compounds have been shown to suppress the growth of Dunning rat prostatic cancer [102]; in addition, it has been shown that the administration of somatostatin analogues with LHRH agonists enhances the inhibitory effect of the LHRH analogues on the growth of experimental prostate tumours [103]. This combination might then improve the clinical response in patients with advanced prostate tumours.

It is not yet known through which mechanisms somatostatin analogues may interfere with the growth of cancer cells. They might act a) by decreasing the release of prolactin, a hormone which is involved in promoting prostatic cell growth [102]; b) by suppressing the secretion of GH involved in prostatic cell growth; and c) by directly inhibiting the mitogenic effects of tissue growth factors. For instance, it has been shown that somatostatin analogues suppress EGF-induced cell replication [102]. In addition, based on the fact that somatostatin analogues block the secretion of the somatomedins which mediate the action of GH and that somatomedin-like peptides are present in prostatic cells and act as mitogenic autocrine factors, it is possible to speculate that somatostatin analogues might interfere with the local production and/or secretion of somatomedins. These possibilities are not necessarily mutually exclusive.

However, further studies are needed to clarify better the link between these factors and the hormonal inputs; these studies might indicate whether other approaches, based on the control of other hormonal signals, could be therapeutically applicable and advantageous compared to the more classical methods already available for the treatment of prostatic tumours.

Acknowledgement

Supported by a grant from the Italian National Research Council (CNR), Special Target Project "Oncology" (contract No. 88;00741; 44), by funds from MPI and by the "Centro di Endocrinologia Oncologica", University of Milan, Italy.

REFERENCES

1 Geller J and Vik Franson A: Endocrine dependent prostate disease. In: Serio M (ed) Perspectives in Andrology. Raven Press, New York 1989 Vol 53 pp 57-69

2 Huggins C, Stevens RE Jr and Hodges CV: Studies on prostatic cancer. II. The effects of castration on advanced carcinoma of the prostate gland. Arch Surg 1941 (43):209-223

3 Vermeulen A: The androgens. In: Grey CH and James VHT (eds) Hormones in Blood. Academic Press, London 1979 Vol 3 pp 355-416

4 Piva F, Motta M and Martini L: Regulation of hypothalamic and pituitary function: long, short, and ultrashort feedback loops. In: DeGroot LJ (ed) Endocrinology. Grume and Stratton, New York 1979 pp 21-33

5 Harper ME, Pike A, Peeling WB and Griffiths K: Steroids of adrenal origin metabolised by human prostatic tissue in vivo and in vitro. J Endocrinol 1974 (60):117-125

6 Labrie F, Dupont A and Belanger A: Complete androgen blockade for the treatment of prostate cancer. In: De Vita VT, Hellman S and Rosenberg SA (eds) Important Advances in Oncology. Lippincott, Philadelphia 1985 pp 193-217

7 Labrie F, Dupont A, Belanger A and St Arnaud R: Treatment of prostate cancer with gonadotropin-releasing hormone agonists. Endocr Rev 1986 (7):67-74

8 Tullner WW: Hormonal factors in the adrenal-dependent growth of the rat ventral prostate. NCI Monogr 1963 (12):211-223

9 Oesterling JE, Epstein JI and Walsh PC: The viability of adrenal androgens to stimulate the adult human prostate: an autopsy evaluation of men with hypogonadotropic hypogonadism and panhypopituitarism. J Urol 1986 (136):1030-1034

10 Krieg M, Bartsh W, Janssen W and Voigt KD: A comparative study of binding metabolism and endogenous levels of androgens in normal hyperplastic and carcinomatous human prostate. J Steroid Biochem 1979 (11) : 615-624

11 Bruchovsky N and Wilson JD: The conversion of testosterone to 5alpha-androstan-17beta-ol-3-one by rat prostate in vivo and in vitro. J Biol Chem 1968 (243):2012-2021

12 Motta M, Zoppi S, Brodie AM and Martini L: Effect of 1,4,6-androstantriene-3,17-dione (ATD),4-hydroxy-4-androstene-3,17-dione (4-OH-A) and 4-acetoxy-4-androstene-3,17-dione (4-Ac-A) on the 5alpha-reduction of androgens in the rat prostate. J Steroid Biochem 1986 (25):593-599

13 Brooks JR, Baptista EM, Berman C, Ham EA, Hichens M, Johnston DBR, Primka RL, Rasmusson GH, Reynolds GF, Schmitt SM and Arth GE: Response of rat ventral prostate to a new and novel 5alpha-reductase inhibitor. Endocrinology 1981 (109):830-836

14 Blohm TR, Laughlin ME and Benson HD: Pharmacological induction of 5alpha-reductase deficiency in the rat: separation of testosterone-mediated and 5alpha-dihydrotestosterone-mediated effects. Endocrinology 1986 (119):959-966

15 Fang S and Liao S: Androgen receptors. Steroid-and-tissue specific retention of 17beta-hydroxy-5alpha-androstan-3-one-protein complex by the cell nuclei of ventral prostate. J Biol Chem 1971 (246):16-24

16 Barrack ER and Coffey DS: The specific binding of estrogens and androgens to the nuclear matrix of sex hormone responsive tissues. J Biol Chem 1980 (255):7265-7275

17 Isaacs JT, Brendler CB and Walsh PC: Changes in the metabolism of dihydrotestosterone in the hyperplastic human prostate. J Clin Endocrinol Metab 1983 (56):139-146

18 Geller J: Benign prostatic hypertrophy: current understanding of its pathogenesis. In: Labrie F and Proulx L (eds) Endocrinology. Excerpta Medica, Amsterdam 1984 pp 909-912

19 Smith CB, Masters JRW and Ghamadian R: Differential androgen metabolism in prostatic tumors. J Endocr 1980 (85):5-6

20 Kirdani RY, Emrich LJ, Pontes EJ, Priore RL and Murphy GP: A comparison of estrogen and androgen receptor levels in human prostatic tissue from patients with non-metastatic and metastatic carcinoma and benign prostatic hyperplasia. J Steroid Biochem 1985 (22):569-575

21 Thompson SA, Rowley DR and Heidger PM: Effects of estrogen upon the fine structure of epithelium and stroma in the rat ventral prostate gland. Invest Urol 1979 (17):83-89

22 Mawhinney MG and Neubauer BL: Actions of estrogen in the male. Invest Urol 1979 (16):409-420

23 Krieg M, Bartsch W, Thomsen M and Voigt KD: Androgens and estrogens: their interaction with stroma and epithelium of human benign hyperplasia and normal prostate. J Steroid Biochem 1983 (19):155-161

24 Ghanadian R and Puah CM: Relationship between oestradiol-17beta, testosterone, dihydrotestosterone and 5alpha-androstane-3alpha, 17beta-diol in human benign hypertrophy and carcinoma of the prostate. J Endocr 1981 (88):255-262

25 Stone NN, Fair WR and Fishman J: Estrogen formation in human prostatic tissue from patients with and without benign prostatic hyperplasia. Prostate 1986 (9):311-318

26 Kaburagi Y, Marino MB, Kirdani RY, Greco JP, Karr JP and Sandberg AA: The possibility of aromatization of androgen in human prostate. J Steroid Biochem 1987 (26):739-742

27 Thorner MO: Prolactin: clinical physiology and the significance and management of hyperprolactinemia. In: Martini L and Besser GM (eds) Clinical Neuroendocrinology. Academic Press, New York 1977 pp 319-361

28 Jacobi GH and Wenderoth UK: New forms and future perspectives in endocrine treatment of prostatic carcinoma. Progress and Controversies in Oncological Urology. Springer, Berlin 1980

29 Aragona C, Bohnet HG and Friesen HG: Localization of prolactin binding in prostate and testis: the role of serum prolactin concentration on

the testicular LH receptor. Acta Endocrin 1977 (84):402-408
30 Jacobi GH: Palliativtherapie des Prostatakarzinoms. Endokrinologische Grundlagen, Klinische Situation, Prolaktinin neues Prinzip. Zuckschwerdt, München 1980
31 Smith C, Assimos D, Lee C and Grayhack JT: Metabolic action of prolactin on the prostate: independent of androgen action. Prostate 1985 (6):49
32 Boyns AR, Griffiths K, Pierrepoint CG and Peeling WB: Prolactin and the prostate. In: Goland M (ed) Normal and Abnormal Growth of the Prostate. Charles C Thomas, Springfield 1975 pp 431-444
33 Manandhar SF and Thomas JA: Effect of prolactin on the metabolism of androgen by the rat ventral prostate gland in vitro. Invest Urol 1976 (14):20-22
34 Farnsworth WE, Slannwhile WR Jr and Sharma M: Interaction of prolactin and testosterone in the human prostate. Urol Res 1977 (15):83-91
35 Berelowitz M, Szabo M, Frohman LA, Firestone S and Chu L: Somatomedin-C mediates growth hormone negative feedback by effects on both the hypothalamus and the pituitary. Science 1981 (212):1279-1281
36 Lostroh AJ and Li CH: Stimulation of sex accessories of hypophysectomised male rat by non-gonadotrophin hormone of the pituitary gland. Acta Endocrin 1975 (25):1-16
37 British Prostate Study Group: Evaluation of plasma hormone concentrations in relation to clinical staging in patients with prostatic cancer. Br J Urol 1979 (51):382-389
38 Sibley PEC, Harper ME, Peeling WB and Griffiths K: Growth hormonal and prostatic tumors: localization using a monoclonal human growth hormone antibody. J Endocr 1984 (103):311-315
39 Wilson EM and Smith EP: Growth factors in the prostate. Prog Clin Biol Res 1987 (239):205-233
40 James R and Bradshaw RA: Polypeptide growth factors. Ann Rev Biochem 1984 (53):259-292
41 Moses HL, Tucker RF, Leof EB, Coffey JR,Halber J and Shipley GD: Type beta transforming growth factor is a growth stimulator and a growth inhibitor. In: Feramisco J, Ozanne B and Stiles C (eds) Cancer Cells. Cold Spring Harbor Laboratory, Cold Spring Harbor 1985 Vol 3 pp 65-74
42 Roberts AB, Anzano MA, Wakefield LM, Roche NS, Stern DF and Sporn MB: Type beta transforming growth factor: a bifunctional regulator of cellular growth. Proc Natl Acad Sci Usa 1985 (82):119-123
43 Nishi N, Matuo Y, Muguruma Y, Yoshitake Y, Nishikawa K and Wada F: A human prostatic growth factor (hPGF): partial purification and characterization. Biochem Biophys Res Commun 1985 (132):1103-1109
44 Story MT, Esch F, Shimasaki S, Sasse J, Jacobs SC and Lawson RK: Amino-Terminal sequence of a large form of basic fibroblast growth factor isolated from human benign prostatic hyperplastic tissue. Biochem Biophys Res Commun 1987 (142):702-709
45 Jinno H, Ueda K, Otaguro K, Kato T, Ito J and Tanaka R: Prostate growth factor in the extracts of benign prostatic hypertrophy. Eur Urol 1986 (12):41-48
46 Nishi N, Matuo Y and Wada F: Partial purification of a major type of rat prostatic growth factor: characterization as an epidermal growth factor-related mitogen. Prostate 1988 (13):209-220
47 Mydlo JH, Bulbul MA, Richon VM, Heston WDW and Fair W: Heparin-binding growth factor isolated from human prostatic extracts. Prostate 1988 (12):343-355
48 Crabb JW, Armes LG, Johnson CM and McKeehan WL: Characterization of multiple forms of prostatropin (prostate epithelial growth factor) from bovine brain. Biochem Biophys Res Commun 1986 (136): 1155-1161
49 Maddy SQ, Chisholm GD, Hawkins RA and Habib FK: Localization of epidermal growth factor receptors in the human prostate by biochemical and immunocytochemical methods. J Endocr 1987 (113):147-153
50 Matuo Y, Nishi N, Matsui S, Sandberg AA, Isaacs JT and Wada F: Heparin binding affinity of rat prostatic growth factor in normal and cancerous prostates: partial purification and characterization of rat prostatic growth factor in the Dunning tumor. Cancer Research 1987 (47):188-192
51 Wilding G, Valverius E, Knabbe C and Gelmann EP: Role of transforming growth factor-alpha in human prostate cancer cell growth. Prostate 1989 (15):1-2
52 Davies P and Eaton CL: Binding of epidermal growth factor by human normal hypertrophic and carcinomatous prostate. Prostate 1989 (14):123-132
53 Nishi N, Matuo Y, Kunitomi K, Takenaka I, Usami M, Kotake T and Wada F: Comparative analysis of growth factors in normal and pathologic human prostates. Prostate 1988 (13):39-48
54 Peehl DM, Wong ST, Bazinet M and Stamey TA: In vitro studies of human prostatic epithelial cells: attempts to identify distinguishing features of malignant cells. Growth Factors 1989 (1):237-250
55 McKeehan WL, Adams PS and Rosser MP: Direct mitogenic effects of insulin, epidermal growth factor, glucocorticoid, cholera toxin, unknown pituitary factors and possibly prolactin, but not androgen on normal rat prostate epithelial cells in serum-free primary cell culture. Cancer Res 1984 (44):1998-2010
56 Fowler JE, Lau JLT, Ghosh L, Mills SE and Mounzer A: Epidermal growth factor and prostatic carcinoma: an immunohistochemical study. J Urol 1988 (139):857-861
57 Traish AM and Wotiz HM: Prostatic epidermal growth factors receptors and their regulation by androgens. Endocrinology 1987 (121):1461-1467
58 Kirdani RY, Muntzing J, Varkarakis JM, Murphy GP and Sandberg AA: Studies on the antiprostatic action of estracyt, a nitrogen mustard of estradiol. Cancer Res 1974 (34):1031-1037
59 Hoisaeter PA: Incorporation of 3H-thymidine into rat ventral prostate in organ culture. Invest Urol 1975 (12):479-483
60 Daehlin L: On the effects of oestrogen in the male. Some effects of different oestrogenic substances in rats and men with prostatic carcinoma. Scand J Urol Nephrol 1985 (91 Suppl):21-35

61 Tan SY, Antonipillai I and Murphy BEP: Inhibition of testosterone metabolism in the human prostate. J Clin Endocrinol Metab 1984 (39):936-941
62 Massa R and Martini L: Interference with the 5alpha-reductase system. Gynec Invest 1972 (2):253-270
63 Jagarinec N and Givner ML: Inhibition of testosterone metabolism of medrogestone in rat ventral prostate in vivo and in vitro. Arch Androl 1981 (7):39-44
64 Martini L and Motta M (eds) Androgens and Antiandrogens. Raven Press, New York 1977
65 Neumann F: Pharmacology and clinical uses of cyproterone acetate. In: Furr BJA and Wakeling AE (eds) Pharmacology and Clinical Uses of Inhibitors of Hormone Secretion and Action. Bailliere Tindall, London 1987 pp 132-159
66 Neri R and Kassen N: Pharmacology and clinical uses of flutamide. In: Furr BJA and Wakeling AE (eds) Pharmacology and Clinical Uses of inhibitors of Hormone Secretion and Action. Bailliere Tindal, London 1987 pp 160-169
67 Raynaud JP, Bonne C, Moguilewsky M, Levebvre FA, Belanger A and Labrie F: The pure antiandrogen RH 23908 (anandron), a candidate of choice for the combined antihormonal treatment of prostatic cancer: a review. Prostate 1984 (5):299-324
68 Neumann F, Habenicht UF and Schacher A: Antiandrogens and target cell response. Different in vivo effects of cyproterone acetate, flutamide and cyproterone. In: McKerns KW, Aakvaag A and Hansson V (eds) Regulation of Target Cell Responsiveness. Plenum Press, New York 1984 Vol 2 pp 489-527
69 Furr BJA: Pharmacological properties and potential clinical utility of ICI 176,334: a novel, non-steroidal, peripherally selective antiandrogen. In: Motta M and Serio M (eds) Hormonal therapy of Prostatic Diseases: Basic and Clinical Aspects. Medicom, Amsterdam 1988 pp 148-161
70 Denis L: A new non-steroidal anti-androgen. In: Murthy JP and Khourys (eds) Therapeutic Progress in Urological Cancers. Alan R Liss Inc, New York 1989 pp 95-103
71 Zoppi S, Cocconi M, Natali A, Costantini A, Serio M, Martini L and Motta M: In vitro effects of an aromatase inhibitor of 5alpha-reductase activity in human hypertrophic prostatic tissue. J Clin Endocrinol Metab 1986 (63):269-271
72 Rasmusson GH: Biochemistry and pharmacology of 5alpha-reductase inhibitors. In: Furr BJA and Wakeling AE (eds) Pharmacology and Clinical Uses of Inhibitors of Hormone Secretion and Action. Bailliere Tindall, London 1987 pp 308-325
73 Wenderoth UK, George FW and Wilson JD: The effect of a 5alpha-reductase inhibitor on androgen-mediated growth of the dog prostate. Endocrinology 1983 (113):569-573
74 Rittmaster RS, Stoner E, Thompson DL, Nance D and Lasseter KC: Effect of MK-906, a specific 5alpha-reductase inhibitor, on serum androgens and androgen conjugates in normal men. J Androl 1989 (10):259-262
75 Habenicht UF, Scwartz K, Schweikert HU, Neumann F and El Etreby MF: Development of a model for the induction of estrogen-related prostatic hyperplasia in the dog and its response to the aromatase inhibitor 4-hydroxy-4-androstene-3,17-dione: preliminary results. Prostate 1986 (8):181-194
76 Baba Y, Matsuo M and Schally AV: Structure of the porcine LH-and FSH-releasing hormone. II. Confirmation of the proposed structure by conventional sequential analyses. Biochem Biophys Res Commun 1971 (44):459-461
77 Karten MJ and Rivier JE: Gonadotropin-releasing hormone analog design. Strucure-function studies toward the development of agonists and antagonists: rationale and perspective. Endocr Rev 1986 (7):44-66
78 Bhasin S and Swerdloff RS: Mechanisms of gonadotropin-releasing hormone agonist action in the human male. Endocr Rev 1986 (7):106-114
79 Schally AV, Comaru-Schally AM and Redding TW: Antitumor effects of analogs of hypothalamic hormones in endocrine-dependent cancers. Proc Soc Exp Biol Med 1984 (175):259-281
80 Clayton RN and Catt KJ: Gonadotropin-releasing hormone receptors: characterization, physiological regulation and relationship to reproductive function. Endocr Rev 1981 (2):186-201
81 Fekete M, Redding TW, Comaru-Schally AM, Pontes JD, Connelly RW, Srkalovic G and Schally AV: Receptors for luteinizing hormone-releasing hormone, somatostatin, prolactin and epidermal growth factor in rat and human prostate cancers and in benign prostate hyperplasia. Prostate 1989 (14):191-208
82 Klign JGM, De Voogt HJ, Schroder FH and De Jong FH: Combined treatment with buserelin and cyproterone acetate in metastatic prostatic carcinoma. Lancet 1985 (2):493
83 Huhtaniemi I, Nikula H and Rannikko S: Treatment of prostatic cancer with a gonadotropin-releasing hormone agonist analog: acute and long term effects on endocrine functions of testis tissue. J Clin Endocrinol Metab 1985 (61):698-704
84 Bouffioux C, Denis L, Mahler C and deLeval J: Le traitement du cancer avancé de la prostate au moyen des analogues de la LHRH: comment prévenir la flambee tumorale (flare-up) initiale possible? Acta Urol Belg 1986 (54):304-308
85 Redding TW, Coy DH and Schally AV: Prostate carcinoma tumor size in rats decreases after administration of antagonists of luteinizing hormone-releasing hormone. Proc Natl Acad Sci USA 1982 (79):1273-1276
86 Hierowski MT, Altamirano P, Redding TW and Schally AV: The presence of LHRH-like receptors in Dunning R-3327 H prostate tumors. Febs Lett 1983 (154):92-96
87 Forti G, Salerno R, Moneti G, Zoppi S, Fiorelli G, Marinoni T, Natali A, Costantini A, Serio M, Martini L and Motta M: Three-month treatment with a long acting gonadotropin-releasing hormone agonist of patients with benign prostatic hyperplasia: effects on tissue androgen concentration, 5alpha-reductase activity and androgen receptor content. J Clin Endocrinol Metab 1989 (68):461-468

88 Geller J, Albert JD, Nachsheim DA and Loza D: Comparison of prostatic cancer tissue dihydrotestosterone levels at the time of relapse following orchiectomy or estrogen therapy. J Urol 1984 (132):693-696

89 Trachtenberg J: Optimal testosterone concentration for the treatment of prostatic cancer. J Urol 1985 (133):888-892

90 Worgul TJ, Santen RJ, Samojlik E, Veldhuis JD, Lipton A, Harvey HA, Drago JR and Rohner TJ: Clinical and biochemical effect of aminoglutethimide in the treatment of advanced prostatic carcinoma. J Urol 1983 (129):51-57

91 Sonino N: The endocrine effects of ketoconazole. J Endocrinol Invest 1986:341-347

92 Kuhn JM, Billebaud T, Navratil H, Moulonguet A et al: Prevention of the transient adverse effects of a gonadotropin-releasing hormone analogue (buserelin) in metastatic prostatic carcinoma by administration of an antiandrogen (nilutamide). N Engl Med 1989 (321):413-418

93 Ahmann FR and Schifman RB: Prospective comparison between serum monoclonal prostate specific antigen and acid phosphatase measurements in metastatic prostatic cancer. J Urol 1987 (137):431-434

94 Navratil H: Double-blind study of anandron versus placebo in stage D2 prostate cancer patients receiving buserelin: results on 49 cases from a multicentre study. In: Murphy GP, Khoury S, Kuss R, Chatelain C and Denis L (eds) Prostate Cancer. Part A: Research, Endocrine Treatment and Histopathology. Progress in Clinical and Biological Research. Vol 243. Alan R Liss, New York 1987 pp 401-410

95 Labrie F, Dupont A, Cusan L, Giguere M et al: Combination therapy with flutamide and castration (LHRH agonist or orchiectomy) in previously untreated patients with clinical stage D2 prostate cancer: Today's therapy of choice. J Steroid Biochem 1988 (30):107-111

96 Crawford ED, Eisenberger MA, Mcleod DG, Spaulding JT et al: A controlled trial of leuprolide with and without flutamide in prostatic carcinoma. N Engl J Med 1989 (321):419-424

97 Schroeder FH, Lock TMTW, Chada DR, Debruyne FMJ et al: Metastatic cancer of the prostate managed with buserelin, versus buserelin plus cyproterone acetate. J Urol 1987 (137):912-917

98 Eighth Congress of the European Association of Urology. London, 18-21 May 1988, Abstracts 42-44

99 Serio M, Costantini A and Di Silverio F: Use of LHRH analogue 'Zoladex' depot alone and with cyproterone acetate in the treatment of advanced prostatic carcinoma. VIII Int Symposium on Future Trends in Chemotherapy, 28-30 March 1988, Tirrenia (Pisa), p 179 (Abstract)

100 Raynaud JP, Namer M and Ojasoo T (eds): Am J Clin Oncol 1988 (11) suppl 2

101 Moreau JP and De Fendis FV: Pharmacological studies of somatostatin and somatostatin-analogues: therapeutic advance and perspectives. Life Sci 1987 (40):419-437

102 Defeudis FV and Moreau JP: Studies on somatostatin analogues might lead to new therapies for certain types of cancer. TIPS 1986 (10):384-386

103 Schally AV and Redding TW: Somatostatin analogs as adjuncts to agonists of luteinizing hormone-releasing hormone in the treatment of experimental prostate cancer. Proc Natl Acad Sci Usa 1987 (84):7275-7279

Oestrogens and Estracyt in Prostate Cancer

Peter Ekman

Department of Urology, Karolinska Hospital, Stockholm, Sweden

At present, oestrogens have limited indications in prostate cancer therapy. In clinical practice, these drugs belong to the past. Since Estracyt is ascribed both oestrogenic and cytotoxic properties, it will be dealt with under a separate heading.

Oestrogens

Historical Background

Our knowledge of the endocrine dependency of the prostate gland goes back to 18th century England, where John Hunter described the atrophy of the prostate and seminal vesicles recorded in bulls following castration [1]. One hundred years later, endocrine manipulation by means of castration for the treatment of BPH had been introduced independently by White in 1895 [2] and by Cabot in 1896 [3]. It soon fell into oblivion, thanks to the introduction of modern prostate surgery, but recently it has received renewed attention [4,5]. The era of endocrine therapy against prostatic disorders started with Charles Huggins, who in the late 1930s, early 1940s, conducted meticulous studies on the endocrine dependency of the prostate gland and the influence - in particular on cancer - of castration, oestrogen and androgen stimulation [6,7]. Less well known is the fact that he was not the first to describe this phenomenon. In 1940 the Swiss urologist Paul Niehaus published a booklet entitled "Prostate Cancer and BPH Are Consequences of Hormonal Imbalance Which Should Be Adjusted, the Sooner the Better. Experience from 13 Years of Cancer Prophylaxis by Means of Hormonal Manipulations" [8]. However, this book contained more speculation than proof regarding the efficacy of hormones against prostatic carcinoma.

Following the pioneering work of Huggins, there was a rapid, world-wide acceptance of endocrine treatment as the more or less ultimate solution to the prostate cancer problem. Endocrine manipulation, either by means of castration or oestrogen substitution, was introduced on a routine basis as standard therapy once the diagnosis was confirmed. In centres with a more aggressive approach, radical surgery was still carried out, albeit in less than 5% of all newly diagnosed cases. In many units in Europe, and perhaps particularly in Scandinavia, oestrogen substitution became the golden rule. In 1966, Charles Huggins was awarded the Nobel Prize for Medicine and Physiology. One year later, the first Veterans Administration study was published, reporting serious cardiovascular side effects from oestrogen treatment [9] and advocating alternative treatment modalities, especially castration.

Efficacy of Oestrogens

Several reports from the late 1960s and early 1970s indicated a direct cytotoxic effect of oestrogens on the cells [10,11]. However, these experiments were based on *in vitro* studies using non-physiological doses of oestrogens. Oestradiol binds to the androgen receptor, but with an affinity of less than one per cent of that of DHT [12]. This means that dosages of approximately 100-150 mg of DES should be used for this effect. Indeed, by raising the doses to these levels in relapsing cases, a short episode of secondary re-

sponse might be registered [13]. Symes and Milroy showed that no cytotoxic effects could be seen *in vitro* when using physiological doses of oestrogens [14].
The most important aspect of oestrogen action is the interference with the pituitary-gonadal axis, reducing LH secretion and bringing androgen production from the testes down to castrate levels [15]. This effect is reached within 10-14 days and remains on these levels as long as the treatment is continued. If treatment lasts for 3 years or more and is then discontinued, serum testosterone may remain on castrate levels for up to another 3 years, despite slowly increasing pituitary gonadal hormones [16]. This is said to indicate a direct effect of the treatment on the Leydig cells [16].
The phenomenon of retained androgen castrate levels is not seen following short-term therapy. Nevertheless, some authors have advocated intermittent oestrogen treatment instead of continuous therapy, treating the patients until good palliation is achieved [17]. The therapy is then stopped until symptoms recur. The rationale for such a treatment modality is an improved quality of life, patients having the opportunity to regain potency and normal mental status during the medicine-free intervals.
A further effect of oestrogens is an increase in sex-hormone-binding globuline (SHBG) levels in the circulation [18]. Not only does SHBG bind the oestrogens, but also the low levels of remaining circulating androgens, making them less well available for the prostate cells. It is, however, not shown that this has any clinical importance favouring oestrogen therapy over surgical castration.

Oestrogenic Drugs

The most widely used preparation for oestrogen therapy is DES, diethylstilboestrol, which can be administered orally in varying doses. In earlier years, often quite high doses were given, 10-20 mg a day, even up to 100 mg as mentioned before, in the hope of a direct cytotoxic effect. The Veterans studies clearly showed that efficient castration levels could be achieved with doses as low as 3 mg or even 1 mg a day, but not with 0.5 or 0.25 mg [9]. The generally recommended dose since then has been 3 mg a day.
In Scandinavia, a parenteral oestrogen preparation, polyoestradiol phosphate (PEP), was tried at a dose of 80 mg on a monthly basis [19]. Since castrate levels were not achieved with this drug, it was combined with a strong oral oestrogen, ethinyl oestradiol, 150 µg/day. In a mixed series of prostate cancer patients, a 5-year survival of 44% was reported in 1963 using PEP alone [19]; with the combination, a 63% 5-year survival was registered in 1971 [20]. This combination has constituted the standard treatment in Scandinavia in all cases of prostate cancer for over a decade.
Other drugs that have been used less frequently include chlorotrianisene (TACE), Honvan (diethylstilboestrol linked to phosherol, in an attempt to increase its cytotoxic effect in the prostate cells), and dienoestrol.

Side Effects of Oestrogen Therapy

The feminising side effects are almost universal. However, gynaecomastia can be prevented by one low dose of radiotherapy (7-10 Gy) to the nipples before treatment is started [21]. The patients are also rendered impotent, may have mental alterations with a tendency to depression and inactivity, and acquire an altered fatty tissue distribution. Some patients suffer from hot flushes. The most serious side effects, though, which have now led to an almost complete withdrawal of oestrogens from the market, are the cardiovascular complications.
As mentioned above, cardiovascular toxicity was first described in the 1967 Veterans report [9], but has since then been confirmed by numerous other investigators [22-24]. Cardiovascular toxicity is most common during the first 6 months. Beyond one year of continuous treatment, such complications are rare [23]. In most series, a frequency of myocardial infarction of 3% is reported. Pulmonary embolism is seen in approximately 4% of patients. Deep vein thrombosis is seen in 4%-5%, cardiac failure in 4%. Peripheral oedema is common, 15%-20%, and cerebrovascular accidents occur in around 2%. In an unselected series of pa-

Table 1. Approximate frequency of cardiovascular complications in an unselected series of patients with prostate cancer treated with oral oestrogens [23]

Complication	Frequency
Thromboembolism	24 %
Ischaemic complications	16 %
Heart failure	29 %
Cerebrovascular events	7 %
Total*	60%

* Several patients had more than one complication simultaneously

tients, reported cardiovascular adverse effects from oestrogens were as high as 60% (Table 1). Pure ischaemic and thromboembolic complications occurred with a frequency of 32%, however, only 8% with a fatal outcome [23].

The major cause of the cardiovascular side effects is a liver-mediated metabolic change. Whereas cholesterol and total serum lipids are hardly affected, a significant increase is seen in the levels of serum triglycerides and in particular the high-density lipoproteins (HDL) [22]. More recently, it has been demonstrated that the cardiovascular toxicity may rather be explained by a liver-induced alteration in coagulation factors [24,25]. The most marked change is an increase in factor VII, but also factor VIII and fibrinogen are increased. A decrease in antithrombin III and an increase in fibrinolysis are also seen, all phenomena that favour venous thromboembolism and vascular ischaemia.

Oestrogen Therapy Without Cardiovascular Toxicity

Interestingly, the parenteral oestrogens seem to exert very little influence on the liver metabolism. As reported by Sotaniemi and Kontturi in 1975 [22], peroral oestrogens led to a significant shift in triglyceride levels, whereas polyoestradiol phosphate did not. This was confirmed recently by a group at Huddinge Hospital, Sweden, using polyoestradiol phosphate in doses up to 320 mg/month [26]. This group also showed that the coagulation factors remained unchanged [27]. This high dose, unlike 160 mg/month, seems to reduce the circulating androgens to castration levels and is, therefore, an interesting treatment alternative when endocrine treatment is considered. In short-term studies the efficacy was similar to castration; long-term studies are under way.

Despite the oral route of administration, the Veterans Administration group [9] were able to show that, by reducing the dose of DES to 1 mg per day, hardly any cardiovascular toxicity was observed, yet the circulating androgen levels were depressed to nearly castrate levels. Large randomised studies on the efficacy of 1 mg DES per day in human prostatic cancer have yet to be carried out.

Controversies

Several controversies exist regarding hormonal treatment of prostatic cancer. A few of them will be discussed briefly.

Can Oestrogens Cure Prostate Cancer?

Prostate cancer is composed of hormone-dependent, hormone-sensitive and hormone-resistant cells [28]. These appear simultaneously in practically all prostate cancers at least at the time of detection, usually with a marked predominance of the hormone-dependent cells. Provided the patient has a cancer consisting exclusively of hormone-dependent cells, he will be "cured" as long as his endocrine suppression lasts. Indeed, it is unlikely that the hormone-dependent prostate cancer cells ever kill the patient; the patient dies from progression of the hormone-independent and hormone-sensitive cells.

Does Endocrine Therapy Prolong Survival?

Numerous reports in the literature indicate that hormone therapy does prolong survival, but almost all of these are based on historical controls [19,20,29,30]. In the paper by Lepor et al. [31], a comparison was made of survival

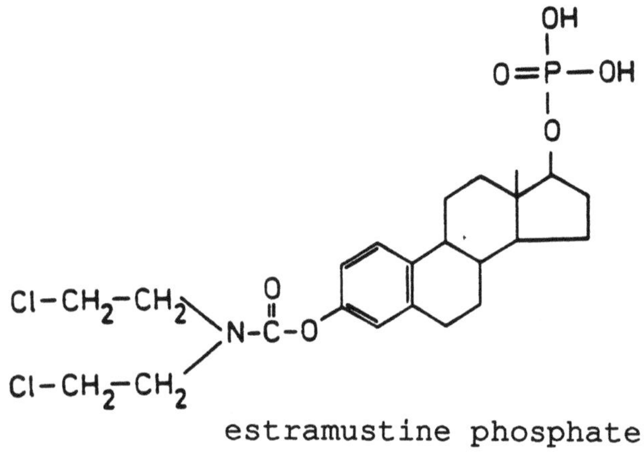

Fig. 1. Structural formula of Estracyt® (estramustine phosphate)

in 100 consecutive patients before 1942, the year when endocrine therapy was introduced at their institution, and 100 consecutive patients following this year. There was, indeed, a statistically significant difference in favour of the hormone-treated group. However, despite the few years of difference between the groups, no difference could be demonstrated when correcting for overall improved survival in the general population, coinciding with the introduction of antibiotics. Numerous investigators failed to prove any difference in survival [32-34], some even believe that, by suppressing the hormone-dependent cells, the hormone-independent cells get more "space" and start growing more rapidly [35].
In conclusion, the matter of timing endocrine treatment will have to wait for randomised studies comparing early versus late endocrine therapy.

Stable Disease

The natural course of prostatic carcinoma is highly unpredictable. Periods of fairly rapid tumour progression may be followed by a complete stabilisation of the process (latent periods). These can occur regardless of presence or absence of treatment. Since such periods cannot be foreseen in any way, the phenomenon severely hampers an adequate interpretation of the results of various forms of treatment. One year after the start of endocrine treatment in advanced prostatic carcinoma, approximately half of the patients will be in "stable disease". The number of these who are true responders can only be a matter of speculation. Hence, this group should be interpreted separately in any treatment protocol.

Estracyt

Estracyt was originally developed as a treatment for breast cancer, based on the hypothesis that a cytotoxic agent bound to a steroid could use the steroid as a carrier to the target, i.e., the specific, hormone-dependent cell. Once there, the cytotoxic agent would be released for more efficient elimination of the cancer cell. The molecule is composed of oestradiol linked to nor-nitrogen mustard via a carbamate bridge (Fig. 1). The phosphate group is attached to the molecule to make it water soluble. After dephosphorylisation in the body, the drug is partly oxidized to estramustine and then further metabolised to oestrone and oestradiol [36]. Approximately 10-15% of the molecule-oestradiol is recovered as free oestradiol and oestrone. With the dosages usually recommended, the amount of oestrogens in the circulation approaches those seen following standard oestrogen treatment [36].
The efficacy of Estracyt against breast cancer was very limited, however. Rat studies revealed that a large amount of radioactive Estracyt was recovered in the rat ventral prostate [37]. Therefore, the drug was tried in human prostate cancer instead and turned out to be at least as effective as conventional oestrogen treatment [38].
The basic concept, i.e., the oestrogen molecule acting as a carrier for the cytotoxic agent, binding to the oestrogen receptor, seems to have limited importance, since human prostatic tissue contains very small amounts of oestrogen receptor [39]. The reason for the marked accumulation of Estracyt in rat prostate is the presence of an excretory protein which binds Estracyt with high capacity and has been called the Estramustine-Binding Protein (EMBP) [40]. This protein constitutes almost 20% of the intracellular protein in rat ventral prostate. The estramustine-binding protein is also present in the hu-

man prostate, albeit in much smaller amounts. This presence allows accumulation of Estracyt in prostate cancer cells providing the possibility to target additional cytotoxic effects from the nor-nitrogen mustard molecule [41].

Mechanism of Action of Estracyt

The mechanism of action of Estracyt is twofold: oestrogenic and cytotoxic. The oestrogenic side effects are similar to those following conventional oestrogen therapy although less frequent. Thromboembolic complications in the Stockholm study were reported to be 13%, as compared to 24% following conventional oestrogen therapy [23].

In recent years, laboratory studies have shown that estramustine is cytotoxic in several human prostate cancer cell lines [42]. The activity was not due to influence on the DNA itself. In studies on the cell line DU 145, it was found that estramustine caused mitotic arrest [43]. After a 24-hour exposure, the chromosomes in metaphase were no longer oriented in the metaphase plane and were also more contracted. This phenomenon is similar to that occurring with treatment with microtubule inhibitors such as colchisine, hence, it was suggested that the cytotoxic action was due to an inhibition of microtubule functions [44]. It was later confirmed that estramustine could, indeed, prevent assembly and cause disassembly of isolated microtubules from the brain via binding to the microtubule-associated proteins [45]. Such proteins are essential for the stability of microtubules. The practical implication of the effect on cytoplasmic microtubules is that these microtubules are responsible for the invasive potential of a cell and, consequently, for the ability to form metastases.

In 1980 it was demonstrated, in a small series of patients, that cytomorphological regression following Estracyt therapy could be noted in 7/10 patients as compared to only 1/10 given conventional oestrogen treatment [46]. By means of cytophotometric microscanning, the same authors discovered that the DNA content of the cancer cells was markedly reduced by Estracyt as compared to standard oestrogen therapy [46].

Clinical Effect of Estracyt

Unfortunately, as mentioned elsewhere in this volume, prostatic carcinoma is not very susceptible to chemotherapy. Therefore, the value of adding a cytotoxic agent in prostate cancer therapy may be questioned. In the following paragraphs, only Estracyt as monotherapy will be discussed. For data on the efficacy of Estracyt in combination with other drugs, the reader is referred to a special chapter on this issue.

As far as primary treatment is concerned, there are 3 major studies worth reporting.

The Stockholm study made an interim report in 1980 [47]. In this study, patients with grade I and II tumours with or without metastases were recruited to receive either the conventional oestrogen treatment, polyoestradiol phosphate plus ethinyl oestradiol, or Estracyt in a dose of 560 to 840 mg/day. A total of 256 patients were enrolled, of whom 150 were evaluable. There was no statistically significant difference in number of responses to treatment, duration of response or response to secondary treatment when a crossover was carried out following relapse. With regard to survival no final evaluation was made [47].

The EORTC study reported their results in 1986 [48]. They compared DES 3 mg/day with Estracyt 280 mg/day. In 227 evaluable patients no difference in response rates, time to progression, or overall survival was recorded.

The third major study, usually called "The Wisconsin Study", was carried out in the US [49]. This was a double-blind, randomised, crossover study only including patients with metastatic disease. The patients were given from 700 up to 1260 mg Estracyt/day depending on body weight. Time to progression in 157 non-castrated patients was significantly in favour of the Estracyt group, however, survival was the same. In the castrated group no difference in time to progression could be noted.

In summary, although the cytotoxic effects were documented *in vitro*, the clinical experience does not seem to confirm any superiority of Estracyt over conventional oestrogen treatment. The Stockholm study has been criticised for including only well and moderately well differentiated cancers - possibly Estracyt is superior in poorly differentiated disease.

Such a study is ongoing but has not yet been evaluated. The EORTC study is criticised for using an exceedingly low dose of the drug. Hence, it is possible that ,by using gram doses of Estracyt as in the Wisconsin series, a longer progression-free survival may be achieved.

Estracyt as Second-Line Therapy

Estracyt therapy as second-line treatment will be discussed elsewhere in this volume. In Scandinavia the drug is used as the first alternative for patients relapsing on endocrine treatment, because of the ease of administration and the relatively few side effects compared to other cytotoxic agents. As in other single or combination chemotherapeutic regimens, about 30% of objective responses are reported, although most of these are stable disease and of short duration.

Summary

- Oestrogen treatment is no longer the first alternative when endocrine therapy is considered.
- Despite its proven cytotoxic efficacy *in vitro*, Estracyt still lacks any proven clinical advantages over standard endocrine therapy, such as castration.
- Polyoestradiol phosphate, parenteral oestrogen, is an interesting treatment alternative, since it is cheap and causes no cardiovascular toxicity.

REFERENCES

1 Hunter J: Observations on the glands situated between the rectum and bladder, called vesiculae seminalis. In: Collected Works of John Hunter, Vol 4. Palmer JF, London 1786 p 31

2 White JW: The results of double castration in hypertrophy of the prostate. Ann Surg 1895 (22):1-80

3 Cabot AT: The question of castration for enlarged prostate. Ann Surg 1896 (24):265-309

4 Schröder FH, Westerhof M, Bosch RJLH and Kurth KH: Benign prostatic hyperplasia treated by castration or the LH-RH analogue buserelin: a report on 6 cases. Eur Urol 1986 (12):318-321

5 Peters CA and Walsh PC: The effect of nafarelin acetate, a luteinizing-hormone releasing hormone agonist, on benign prostatic hyperplasia. N Engl J Med 1987 (317):599-604

6 Huggins C and Hodges CV: Studies on prostatic cancer. I. The effect of castration, of estrogen and of androgen injection on serum phosphatases in metastatic carcinoma of the prostate. Cancer Res 1941 (1):293-297

7 Huggins C, Stevens RE Jr and Hodges CV: Studies on prostatic cancer. II. The effects of castration on advanced carcinoma of the prostate gland. Arch Surg 1941 (43):209-223

8 Niehaus P: Prostata-Krebs wie Paraprostata-Hypertrophie sind Folgen hormonaler Störungen, die wir je früher je besser beeinflussen können. Med Verlag H Huber, Bern 1940 pp 13-48

9 Veterans Administration Cooperative Urological Research Group: Treatment and survival of patients with cancer of the prostate. Surg Gynecol Obstet 1967 (124):1011-1017

10 Farnsworth WE: A direct effect of estrogens on prostatic metabolism of testosterone. Invest Urol 1969 (6):423-427

11 Harper ME, Fahmy AR, Pierrepoint CG and Griffiths K: The effect of some stilboestrol components on DNA polymerase from human prostatic tissue. Steroids 1970 (15):89-103

12 Snochowski M, Pousette Å, Ekman P, Bression D, Andersson L, Högberg B and Gustafsson JÅ: Characterization and measurement of the androgen receptor in human benign prostatic hyperplasia and prostatic carcinoma. J Clin Endocrinol Metab 1977 (45):920-930

13 Fergusson JD and Franks LM: Response of prostatic carcinoma to oestrogen treatment. Br J Surg 1953 (40):422-428

14 Symes EK and Milroy EJG: An experimental approach to the optimum oestrogen dosage in prostatic carcinoma. Br J Urol 1978 (50):562-566

15 Jönsson G, Olsson AM, Luttrop W, Cekan Z, Purvis K and Diczfalusy E: Treatment of prostatic carcinoma with various types of estrogen derivatives. In: Munson PL, Diczfalusy E, Glover J and Olson RE (eds) Endocrine Control of the Prostate. Academic Press, New York, Vitamins and Hormones 1975 (33): 351-376

16 Tomic R and Bergman B: Hormonal effects of cessation of estrogen treatment for prostatic carcinoma. J Urol 1987 (138):801-803

17 Klotz LH, Herr HW, Morse MJ and Whitmore WF Jr: Intermittent endocrine therapy for advanced prostate cancer. Cancer 1986 (58):2546-2550

18 Stege R, Fröhlander N, Carlström K, Pousette Å and von Schoultz B: Steroid sensitive proteins, growth hormone and somatomedin C in prostatic cancer: effects of parenteral and oral estrogen therapy. Prostate 1987 (10):333-338

19 Jönsson G, Diczfalusy E, Plantin LO, Röhl L and Birke G: Estradurin (polyestradiol phosphate) in the treatment of prostatic carcinoma: a clinical and steroid metabolic study. Acta Endocrinol 1963 (44 Auppl 83):1-41

20 Jönsson G: Treatment of prostatic carcinoma combined with ethinylestradiol. Scand J Urol Nephrol 1971 (5):97-102

21 Larsson LG and Sundbom CM: Roentgen irradiation of the male breast. Acta Radiol 1962 (58):253-256

22 Sotaniemi EA and Kontturi MJ: Serum lipid levels and thromboembolic complications during estrogen therapy of prostatic cancer. Scand J Urol Nephrol 1975 (9):89-93

23 Hedlund PO, Gustafsson H and Sjögren S: Cardiovascular complications to treatment of prostatic cancer with estramustine phosphate (Estracyt®) or conventional estrogen. A follow-up of 212 randomized patients. Scand J Urol Nephrol 1980 (Suppl 55):103-105

24 Henriksson P, Blombäck M, Bratt G, Edhag O, Eriksson A and Vesterqvist O: Effects of oestrogen therapy and orchidectomy on coagulation and prostanoid synthesis in patients with prostatic cancer. Med Oncol & Tumour Pharmacother 1989 (6):219-225

25 Blombäck M, Hedlund PO and Säwe U: Changes in blood coagulation and fibrinolysis in patients on different treatment regimens for prostatic cancer. Predictors for cardiovascular complications? Thromb Res 1986 (44):783-791

26 Stege R, Carlström K, Collste L, Eriksson A, Henriksson P, Pousette Å and von Schoultz B: Single-drug parenteral estrogen treatment in prostatic cancer: a study of two maintenance-dose regimens. Prostate 1988 (49):111-121

27 Henriksson P, Blombäck M, Eriksson A, Stege R and Carlström K: Effects of parenteral oestrogen on the coagulation system in patients with prostatic carcinoma. Br J Urol (in press)

28 Isaacs JT and Coffey DS: Adaptation versus selection as the mechanism responsible for the relapse of prostatic cancer to androgen ablation as studied in the Dunning R-3327-H adenocarcinoma. Cancer Res 1981 (41):5070-5075

29 Nesbit RM and Baum WC: Endocrine control of prostatic carcinoma. Clinical and statistical survey of 1818 cases. J Amer Med Assoc 1950 (143):1317-1320

30 Pollen JJ: Endocrine treatment of prostatic cancer. Urology 1983 (21):555-559

31 Lepor H, Ross A and Walsh PC: The influence of hormonal therapy on survival of men with advanced prostatic cancer. J Urol 1982 (128):335-340

32 Javadpour N: Endocrine treatment of disseminated prostatic cancer. In: Javadpour N (ed) Principles and Management of Urological Cancer. Williams and Wilkins, Baltimore 1983 (II) pp 409-416
33 Blackard CE, Byar DP, Jordan WP and the Veterans Administration Cooperative Urological Research Group: Orchiectomy for advanced prostatic cancer: a re-evaluation. Urology 1973 (1):553-560
34 Parker MC, Cook A, Riddle PR, Fryatt I, O'Sullivan J and Shearer RJ: Is delayed treatment justified in carcinoma of the prostate? Br J Urol 1987 (57):724-728
35 Grossman BH: Hormonal therapy of prostatic carcinoma: is there a rationale for delayed treatment? Urology 1986 (27):199-204
36 Gunnarsson PO, Plym-Forshell G, Fritjofsson Å and Nilsson SB: Plasma concentrations of estramustine phosphate and its major metabolites in patients with prostatic carcinoma treated with different doses of estramustine phosphate. Scand J Urol Nephrol 1981 (15):201-206
37 Plym-Forshell G and Nilsson H: The distribution of radioactivity after administration of labelled estramustine phosphate (Estracyt®), estradiol-17ß-phosphate, and estradiol to rats. Acta Pharmacol et Toxicol 1974 (35 Suppl 1):28-33
38 Jönsson G and Högberg B: Treatment of advanced prostatic carcinoma with Estracyt: a preliminary report. Scand J Urol Nephrol 1971 (5):103-107
39 Ekman P, Barrack ER, Greene GL, Jensen EV and Walsh PC: Estrogen receptors in human prostate: Evidence for multiple binding sites. J Clin Endocrinol Metab 1983 (57):166-176
40 Forsgren B, Högberg B, Gustafsson JÅ and Pousette Å: Binding of estramustine, a nitrogen mustard derivative of estradiol-17ß, in cytosol from rat ventral prostate. Acta Pharmaceut Suec 1978 (15):23-32
41 Norlen BJ, Andersson SB, Björk P, Gunnarsson PO and Fritjofsson Å: Uptake of estramustine phosphate (Estracyt) metabolites in prostatic cancer. J Urol 1988 (140):1058-1062
42 Müntzing J, Jensen G and Högberg B: Pilot study on the growth inhibition by estramustine phosphate (Estracyt) of rat mammary tumours sensitive and insensitive to oestrogens. Acta Pharmacol et Toxicol 1979 (44):1-6
43 Hartley-Asp B: Estramustine induced mitotic arrest in two human prostatic cell lines DU 145. Prostate 1984 (5):93-100
44 Wallin M, Deinum J and Fridén B: Interaction of estramustine phosphate with microtubule-associated proteins. FEBS Lett 1985 (179):289-293
45 Kanje M, Deinum J, Wallin M, Ekström P, Edström A and Hartley-Asp B: The effect of estramustine phosphate on the assembly of isolated brain microtubules and fast axonal transport. Cancer Res 1985 (45):2334-2339
46 Leistenschneider W and Nagel R: Estracyt therapy of advanced prostatic cancer with special reference to control of therapy with cytology and DNA cytophotometry. Eur Urol 1980 (6):111-115
47 Andersson L, Berlin T, Boman J, Collste L, Edsmyr F, Esposti PL, Gustafsson H, Hultgren L, Hedlund PO, Leander G, Nordle Ö, Norlen H and Tillegård P: Estramustine versus conventional estrogenic hormones in the initial treatment of highly and moderately differentiated prostatic carcinoma: a randomized study. Scand J Urol Nephrol 1980 (Suppl 55):143-145
48 Smith PH, Suciu S and Robinson MRG, Richards B, Bastable JRG, Glashan RW, Bouffioux C, Lardennois B, Williams RE, de Pauw M and Sylvester R: A comparison of the effect of diethylstilbestrol with low dose estramustine phosphate in the treatment of advanced prostatic cancer: final analysis of a phase III trial of the European Organization for Research on Treatment of Cancer. J Urol 1986 (136):619-623
49 Benson RC and Gill GM: Estramustine phosphate compared with diethylstilbestrol. A randomized, double-blind, crossover trial for stage D prostate Cancer. Am J Clin Oncol 1986 (9):341-351

Antiandrogens in the Treatment of Prostate Cancer

Fritz H. Schröder

Department of Urology, Erasmus University and Academic Hospital, P.O. Box 1738, 3000 DR Rotterdam, The Netherlands

Endocrine management of human prostatic carcinoma remains a controversial issue because of a number of unanswered questions. Such questions are: Is there an optimal endocrine treatment? What is the best time to start endocrine treatment? Is it advantageous for our patients to exclude not only testicular but also adrenal androgens (total androgen suppression)? Does endocrine treatment prolong life? What is the best way to achieve proper palliation of long duration?

The issue of the use of antiandrogens is closely related to many of these points of discussion. Antiandrogens are suitable to counteract testicular as well as adrenal androgens. Pure antiandrogens as monotherapy, while leading to an increase of plasma testosterone, may still exert tumour control while preserving potency in most patients treated in such a way. The clinician who is dealing with prostate cancer in his daily practice has to have some basic knowledge about these substances which are used with increasing frequency. It is the goal of this chapter to supply proper knowledge for clinical use, to point out side effects and limitations and to define the role of antiandrogens in daily management of prostate cancer.

Definitions and Structure of Antiandrogens

Antihormones in general can be defined as substances that are able to counteract exogenous hormones after exclusion of the corresponding hormone source from the organism. The classical model for antiandrogens, the ventral prostate of the rat, shrinks after castration. If the rat is then treated with an androgen, the original volume of the prostate can be restituted. This restitution can be effectively counteracted by antiandrogens, the model can be used and has been used to study the effectiveness and potency of such substances.

Some antiandrogens, in addition to their effectiveness at the target cell level, also have antigonadotropic properties. According to their structure, these are called steroidal antiandrogens of the cyproterone acetate (CPA) type. Antiandrogens which do not interfere with the pituitary gonadal axis are called pure antiandrogens. Some of these are steroidal. Most other compounds are structurally similar to flutamide (FLU), the oldest and best studied substance in this group. The structural formulas of cyproterone actetate and flutamide are indicated in Figure 1.

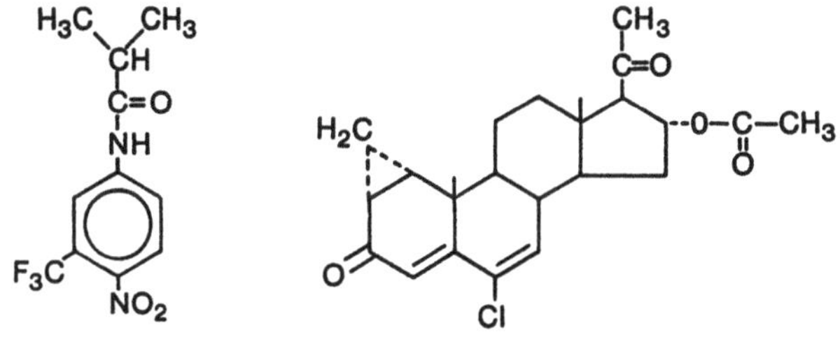

Flutamide Cyproteroneacetate

Fig. 1. Structural formulas of cyproterone acetate (CPA) and flutamide, examples of steroidal and non-steroidal antiandrogens

Mechanisms of Action of Pure and Steroidal Antiandrogens

Extensive reviews of the properties of these substances have recently been presented by Schröder [3], Jacobi and Neumann [4] and Furr [5].

Target cells for androgens are located in many areas of the animal and human bodies and it is believed that steroid hormones exert their action exclusively through specific nuclear receptor systems which are only present in target cells. Target cells are located in all areas that in some way depend on androgens: the male genital skin, male hair follicles, the epididymis and spermatic ducts, the seminal vesicles, the prostate, fatty tissues, male and female breast tissue, etc. However, androgen target cells are also located in the hypothalamic area of the diencephalon where luteinising hormone-releasing hormone (LHRH) is produced under the regulation of a negative feed-back mechanism governed by steroid hormones, including androgens. The effects of antiandrogens must be seen as the simultaneous action of these substances on all target cells.

Some of the effects of pure and steroidal antiandrogens are summarised in Table 1. The impact on endocrine and endocrine response parameters in the intact rat very clearly illustrates the differences between pure and steroidal antiandrogens. Plasma testosterone and dihydrotestosterone (DHT) rise with a pure antiandrogen because these substances inhibit the negative diencephalic feed-back, lead to an increase in LHRH and subsequently LH and testosterone production and Leydig cell hyperplasia. Steroidal antiandrogens lead to a decrease in the same parameters because, in addition to their antiandrogenic activity, they may act as gestagens and as such decrease LHRH and LH as well as testosterone production. Testosterone is the substrate for 5-alpha-reduction resulting in DHT and for aromatisation, which is responsible for male oestrogen production. Plasma DHT, with the pure antiandrogen, increases because of an increase of the rate of these 2 processes which are substrate dependent. With the use of a steroidal antiandrogen, DHT and E2 decrease because there is less circulating testosterone. With the use of a pure antiandrogen, there will be a limit to the rise of plasma testosterone because, at a given moment, rising testosterone and E2 levels will activate the normal diencephalic negative feed-back mechanism, which will then shut off testosterone production by the Leydig cells.

Table 1. Effects of pure and steroidal antiandrogens (AA) on endocrine parameters in intact male rats

Parameters	Pure AA	Steroidal AA
Plasma T	rise	decrease
Plasma DHT	rise	decrease
Plasma E2	rise	decrease
LH	rise	decrease
FSH	rise	decrease
Ventral prostate wt.	decrease	decrease
Seminal vesicle wt.	decrease	decrease
Leydig cells	hyperplasia	atrophy
Prolactine	same	same
Adrenal androgens	same	same
Libido + potency	maybe preserved	impotent

T = Testosterone DHT = 5-alpha-dihydrostestosterone
E2 = Oestradiol LH = luteotropic hormone
FSH = follicle stimulating hormone

source: Knuth et al. [1], Carlström et al. [2]

In the intact animal, with both substances in short-term experiments, a decrease of the weight of target organs such as the ventral prostate and seminal vesicles results. In the case of a pure antiandrogen of the flutamide type, this is due to the direct action at the target cell level. As time goes on, it would be logical that this effect is overruled by increasing androgen levels. However, stimulation of target organs after longer periods of time does not seem to occur in all species. In this respect, the mechanism of pure antiandrogens is still poorly understood. With a steroidal antiandrogen target organ, weights in intact animals will decrease in a more pronounced fashion because of the combination of 2 factors: the lowering of plasma testosterone and the antiandrogenic effect of these substances. Prolactin and adrenal androgen levels are not effected by either substance.

This background information is important for the understanding of the use of antiandrogens in humans. However, there is evidence, and this will be presented later on, that the rise of plasma testosterone resulting in humans with the use of flutamide is self-limiting. The potency of antiandrogens is best studied in castrated rats which are subsequently supplemented with exogenous androgen. In such experiments, it has been shown by Neri et al. [6] that flutamide is roughly twice as strong an antiandrogen as cyproterone acetate. He has also shown that this difference can be compensated by dosage.

Pharmacological Properties of Available Antiandrogens

At this moment, there are only 3 antiandrogens available for clinical use. These substances have been approved in some countries but not in all. Only these 3 drugs, cyproterone acetate (CPA), flutamide (FLU) and nilutamide (NIL), will be dealt with in this context.

Cyproterone Acetate

Cyproterone acetate is a steroidal antiandrogen with antigonadotropic effects. The properties of cyproterone acetate have been extensively described by Neumann et al. in 1984 [7] and in earlier publications by the same author. CPA has approximately half the antiandrogenic potency of FLU, it is also a gestagen and has antigonadotropic activity. The substance is well resorbable and has a short plasma half-life, necessitating t.i.d. dosage. In humans, CPA has very few side effects besides loss of libido and potency, which are inherent to its mechanism of action. Occasional disturbances of liver function have been described. Hot flushes and gynaecomastia are not usually seen with CPA.
The recommended dose for human use is 100 mg every 8 hours. This dose is required if CPA is used as monotherapy. In combination with castration or other principles that exclude testicular androgen production, a much lower dose can be applied. 50 mg t.i.d. has been recommended by the company and has been used in EORTC Genito-Urinary Group study 30843 and other protocols. Probably, an even lower dose is sufficient to suppress adrenal androgens. This dose is not known and is very difficult to determine.
CPA has been extensively used in clinical routine and in phase II and phase III studies. It has been found to be equally active as standard methods of treatment such as castration or low dose diethylstilboestrol (DES). This will be referred to later on in this chapter.

Flutamide

Flutamide is a potent pure antiandrogen with a plasma half-life of 5 to 6 hours. This again necessitates t.i.d. use. Flutamide is reduced to hydroxyflutamide after resorption. Hydroxyflutamide is the active metabolite. The substance has peripheral and central activity on all androgen target cells. It has no antigonadotropic properties. Flutamide is excreted by the kidneys. Human toxicity includes those symptoms reported by DeKernion et al. in 1988 [8] as moderate and severe in respective percentages: nausea (34%, 12%), anorexia (38%, 23%), diarrhoea (15%, 6%), cardiovascular (6%, 5%), oedema (18%, 5%). Cardiovascular symptoms may not be specific side effects of flutamide. In addition to the symptoms noted by DeKernion et al., Lundgren [9] and McFarlane et al. [10] noted gynaecomastia, impotence, depression, dizziness and hot flushes. Severe hepatic toxicity, which is reversible after discontinuation of treatment, has been described in a few cases.
The recommended dose of flutamide is 250 mg t.i.d. Dose recommendations do not differ for monotherapy and combination regimens aiming at total androgen suppression. Determination of the dose of pure antiandrogen in the human situation remains a serious problem because of the kinetics of androgen production under treatment. The problem will, again, be addressed later on in this chapter.
Flutamide has been applied clinically on a broad scale. No controlled trials of sufficient size, however, are available to establish its effectiveness as monotherapy. Such trials are desirable because of the potential of flutamide to preserve potency in previously potent men. In combination treatment with LHRH analogues, flutamide has been used effectively to counteract adrenal androgens (total

androgen suppression, total androgen blockade).

Nilutamide (NIL, Anandron)

Nilutamide, which is structurally closely related to flutamide, has a half-life in plasma of 45 hours. The substance is well resorbed. Because of these properties, NIL can be used once a day. Human toxicity includes hot flushes, nausea, vomiting, visual disturbances, alcohol intolerance in some patients and, rarely, interstitial pneumonitis. Monotherapy is not recommended because of the uncertainties which concern the subsequent rise of plasma testosterone. The dose in combination treatments is recommended to be 300 mg per day. NIL can be used after castration or in combination with LHRH agonists or antangonists or other principles which suppress testicular androgen production. The characteristics of NIL have recently been completely reviewed by Ojasoo [11]. NIL has been extensively used in randomised and non-randomised prospective clinical studies. It is assumed to be equally effective as FLU. Clinical studies with NIL for this reason will not be discussed separately in detail.

A new, potent, long-acting antiandrogen, casodex, has recently been described by Furr [5]. This substance has a long half-life in plasma of 5 to 7 days, it is well resorbed and 5 to 10 times more potent than FLU in rat studies. The substance is not yet available for clinical use and will therefore not be further discussed in this context.

Dosage Problems and Specific Side Effects of Antiandrogens

The determination of the proper dosage of antiandrogens remains a difficult problem. Levels of steroids and other hormones in plasma do not give a clue as to the proper suppression of androgenic activity at the target cell level. It has been shown that cyproterone acetate prevents the translocation of the androgen receptor and of the conjugated steroid hormone into the nucleus by Brinkman and co-workers [12]. This was, however, not confirmed by other authors. It has recently become possible to study directly the response of the target organ, human prostate and human prostate carcinoma by means of volume determinations through transrectal ultrasound or by means of determining the proliferation index of these tumours with the Ki-67 marker as described by Gallee [13]. Unfortunately, such techniques, which in a sensitive way will allow to determine response at the target organ in a time-course fashion, have not been applied yet to the use of pure antiandrogens. The study of the response of serum markers such as prostate specific antigen (PSA) also needs to be undertaken in controlled situations. The problem of those findings especially exists for the use of pure antiandrogens in monotherapy, where it is necessary to compensate for rising plasma testosterone.

It is possible that a number of specific symptoms which are seen with the use of pure antiandrogens in monotherapy are due to the rising plasma testosterone. These include the maintenance of libido and potency, the occurrence of gynaecomastia and hot flushes.

The possible explanations for the persistence of libido and potency under flutamide treatment include the possibility that rising plasma testosterone values maintain potency. In the author's view, the routine clinical use of pure antiandrogens as monotherapy should be restricted until clear evidence is presented that elevation of plasma testosterone values, which occur under flutamide treatment and which probably maintain potency, do not also stimulate tumour growth.

Lund and Rasmussen [14] recently studied plasma testosterone under flutamide treatment for the duration of one year. It turned out that its levels rise to a maximum of about 1.5 times normal values at 6 months and that subsequently a slow decrease occurs. This decrease is unexplained. One possible explanation is that the rising oestrogenic activity together with the rising testosterone triggers the normal negative feed-back. Rising oestrogen levels also are the most likely cause of gynaecomastia. The pathogenesis of hot flushes has recently been studied by Radlmaier [15]. It can be explained by the pulsatile release of gonadotrophins which, in excess, stimulate catecholamine production. Catecholamines are involved in temperature regulation. The role of gonadotrophins in this process also explains why hot flushes can be effectively treated with CPA, as was shown by Eaton and McGuire [16].

Antiandrogens in the Treatment of Prostate Cancer

Since total androgen suppression will be a separate issue within this monograph, the combination treatment will be excluded from this review, which will concentrate on monotherapy with cyproterone acetate and flutamide.

Cyproterone Acetate

Cyproterone acetate has been shown in prospective randomised trials to be equally effective as 3 mg of DES by Pavone et al. [17], to castration by Varenhorst [18], and to oestradiol undecylate 100 mg i.m. per month by Jacobi et al. [19]. De Voogt et al. [20] found that cardiovascular symptoms were significantly less with cyproterone acetate 250 mg/day as compared to 3 mg of DES/day. Other side effects of CPA which are not related to the mechanism of action are rare. Cyproterone acetate today must be considered an alternative mode of standard treatment of metastatic prostatic carcinoma as monotherapy. It has the potential advantage of also counteracting adrenal androgens and thus achieving total androgen suppression without combination with other substances.

Flutamide

Flutamide alone unfortunately has not been studied in a sufficiently large and well conducted randomised phase III study in comparison to standard treatment. Phase II information is available and is reviewed in Table 2. Most studies are small, follow up is usually limited to less than one year. Besides a large number of small studies, there are 2 larger studies by Sogani and Whitmore [27] and Neri and Kassem [28]. Sogani and Whitmore have carried out a careful phase II study which includes a separate evaluation of a large number of subjective and objective parameters for response and progression such as bone pain, decrease in serum acid phosphatase, change in prostatic volume, improvement of hydronephrosis, improvement of soft tissue metastases, voiding symptoms and improvement of the general condition. The results are impressive and show response rates between 70% and 90% for most parameters, including the soft-tissue metastases. Pre-existent hydronephrosis showed the poorest response and disappeared only in 5 of 11 cases. The authors conclude that flutamide is effective as monotherapy. Unfortunately, they do not present long-term results. The protocol continued until relapse, which occurred between 2 and 56 months after initiation, with an average of 12.5 months. Unfortunately, plasma testosterone values at the time of relapse are not avail-

Table 2. Results of clinical studies of flutamide monotherapy in untreated M1 patients

Author	No.pts.	Treatment duration	Response	
Irwin [21]	12	3 months	8	
Stoliar [22]	1	3-39 weeks	7	
Prout [23]	13	2-20 months	7	
Jacobo [24]	13	12-38 weeks	5	
Airhart [25]	20	12 weeks	8	
Narayana [26]	11	?	0	
Sogani [27]	72	12.5 months	49	(68%)
Neri [28]	81	25-36 months	37	(46%)
Lundgren [29]	10	> 9 months	2	

able. Neri and Kassem compared the daily dose of 750 mg in 39 patients to 1500 mg in 42 patients. They found a slightly higher rate of response with the higher dosage. The differences were, however, not statistically significant. Response was studied according to the criteria of the National Prostatic Cancer Project (NPCP). Partial responses occurred in 28% and 38% of cases, respectively.

Two phase III studies are available, which compare flutamide to standard forms of treatment. Unfortunately, both studies are not large enough and have not reached the duration of follow up that would be necessary to show comparative effectiveness of flutamide. Neri and Kassem [28] compared 750 mg and 1500 mg of flutamide per day to 1 mg of DES per day. There was a difference in mean survival time in favour of the flutamide group. This difference was, however, not significant. The study is insufficient to establish the effectiveness of flutamide in comparison to 1 mg of DES. Lund and Rasmussen [14] compared 3 mg of DES to 750 mg of flutamide per day. This study was prospective and randomised, 20 patients were recruited to each arm. Follow up amounts to one year. No differences in response and progression rates were seen. Plasma testosterone values were determined every 3 months and have already been referred to earlier in this chapter. The fact that all patients who were potent prior to entry also remained potent during flutamide treatment is an important prospective. Still, the effectiveness of flutamide as monotherapy needs to be established in a proper phase III trial in comparison to standard treatment.

Early Treatment with Pure Antiandrogens as Monotherapy

Flutamide has been used as monotherapy in localised prostatic cancer either with the purpose to shrink the primary tumour or based on the assumption that early endocrine management is superior to its delay. In both instances, no clinical proof is available at this time. The issue of adjuvant endocrine treatment has been recently reviewed by Bosch et al. [29]. Since the information available in the literature is not conclusive, this problem is presently subject to clinical research. It can be expected that early endocrine treatment will delay progression but will not contribute to a prolongation of life or an improvement of the cancer-related death rate. Endocrine treatment of locally confined prostatic carcinoma should be limited to patients who are not eligible to potentially curative management, especially if obstruction is present and, in all other more elective clinical situations, to prospective clinical studies.

REFERENCES

1 Knuth UA, Hano R, Nieschlag E: Effect of Flutamide or Cyproterone Acetate on pituitary and testicular hormones in normal men. J Clin Endocrinol Metab 1984 (59):963-969
2 Carlström K, Pousette A, Stege R: Basal and ACTH-stimulated adrenal steroids in prostatic cancer patients during treatment with LH-RH analogue and Flutamide. Urol Res 1989 (17-5) Abstract 52:339
3 Schröder FH: Antiandrogenic substances in the management of prostatic cancer. In: Beck et al (eds) Recent Results in Cancer Research 118. Hormone-Related Malignant Tumors. Springer-Verlag, Berlin 1990 (in press)
4 Jacobi GH, Neumann F: The case for Cyproterone acetate. Bailliere's Clin Oncol 1988 (2-3):571-580
5 Furr BJA: The case for pure antiandrogens. Bailliere's Clin Oncol 1988 (2-3):581-590
6 Neri RO, Florance K, Koziol P, Cleave S van: A biological profile of a nonsteroidal antiandrogen, SCH 13521 (4'-Nitro3'-Trifluoromethylisobutyranilide). Endocrinol 1972 (91):427-37
7 Neumann F, Habenicht UF, Schacher A: Antiandrogens and target cell response - different in vivo effects of cyproterone acetate, flutamide and cyproterone. In: McKerns W, Aakvaag A, Hansson V (eds) Regulation of Target Cell Responsiveness 2. Plenum Press, New York 1984 pp 489-527
8 DeKernion JB, Murphy GP, Priore R, Investigators of National Prostatic Cancer Project: Comparison of Flutamide and Emcyt in hormone-refractory metastatic prostatic cancer. Urology 1988 (21-4):312-317
9 Lundgren R: Flutamide as primary treatment for metastatic prostatic cancer. Br J Urol 1988 (59)156-158
10 MacFarlane JR, Tolley DA: Flutamide therapy for advanced prostatic cancer: a phase II study. Br J Urol 1985 (57):172-174
11 Ojasoo T: Nilutamide. Drugs of the Future 1987 (12-8):763-770
12 Brinkmann AO, Lindh LM, Breedveld DI, Mulder E, Molen HJ van der: Cyproterone Acetate prevents translocation of the androgen receptor in the rat prostate. Mol Cell Endocrinol 1983 (32):117-129
13 Gallee MPW, Steenbrugge GJ van, Kate FJW ten, Schröder FH, Kwast ThH van der: Determination of the proliferative fraction of a transplantable hormone dependent, human prostatic carcinoma (PC-82) by monoclonal antibody Ki-67: potential application for hormone therapy monitoring. JNCI 1987 (79):1333
14 Lund F, Rasmussen F: Flutamide versus Stilbestrol in the management of advanced prostatic cancer. Br J Urol 1988 (61):140-142.
15 Radlmaier A, Bormacher K, Neumann F: Hot flushes: mechanism and prevention. In: Schröder FH (ed) EORTC Genitourinary Group Monograph 8: Treatment of Prostatic Cancer: Facts and Controversies. Alan R Liss, New York 1990 (in press)
16 Eaton AC, McGuire N: Cyproterone Acetate in treatment of post-orchidectomy hot flushes. Double blind cross over trial. The Lancet 1983 (8363):1336-1337
17 Pavone-Macaluso M, Voogt HJ de, Viggiano G, Barasolo B, Lardennoi B, Pauw M de, Sylvester R and members of the EORTC GU Group: Comparison of Diethylstilbestrol and Cyproterone acetate and Medroxyprogesterone acetate in the treatment of advanced prostatic cancer: final analysis of a phase III trial of the EORTC Urological Group. J Urol 1986 (136):624-631
18 Varenhorst E: Metabolic changes during endocrine treatment in carcinoma of the prostate. A prospective study in man with special reference to cardiovascular complications during treatment with estrogens, or Cyproterone acetate or after orchiectomy. Thesis, Linköping University, 1980
19 Jacobi GH, Altwein JE, Kurth KH, Basting R, Hohenfellner R: Treatment of advanced prostatic cancer with parenteral Cyproterone acetate. A phase III randomized trial. Br J Urol 1980 (52):208-215
20 Voogt HJ de, Smith PH, Pavone-Macaluso M et al: Cardiovascular side effects of Diethylstilbestrol, Cyproterone acetate, Medroxyprogesterone acetate and Estramustine phosphate used for the treatment of advanced prostatic cancer: results from EORTC trials 30761 and 30762. J Urol 1986 (135):303-307
21 Irwin RJ, Prout GJ, Jr.: A new antiprostatic agent for treatment of prostatic carcinoma. Surgical Forum 1973 (24):536-538
22 Stoliar B, Albert DJ: SCH 13521 in the treatment of advanced carcinoma of the prostate. J Urol 1974 (111):803-807
23 Prout GR, Irwin RJ, Kliman B, Daly JJ, MacLaughin RA, Griffin PP: Prostatic cancer and SCH 13421. II Histological and pituitary gonadal axis. J Urol 1975 (113):834-840
24 Jacobo E, Schmidt JD, Weinstein SH, Flocks RH: Comparison of Flutamide (Sch 13521) and Diethylstilbestrol in untreated advanced prostatic cancer. Urology 1976 (8):231-233
25 Airhart RA, Barnett TF, Sullivan JW, Levie RL, Schlegel JU: Flutamide therapy for carcinoma of the prostate. South Med J 1978 (71):798-801
26 Narayana AS, Loening SA, Culp DA: Flutamide in the treatment of metastatic carcinoma of the prostate. Br J Urol 1981 (53):152-153
27 Sogani PC, Vagaiwala MR, Whitmore WF: Experience with Flutamide in patients with advanced prostatic cancer without prior endocrine therapy. Cancer 1984 (54):774-750
28 Neri RO, Kassem N: Biological and clinical properties of antiandrogens. In Bresciani F et al (eds) Progress in Cancer Research and Therapy 31. Raven Press, New York 1984 pp 507-518
29 Bosch R, Schröder FH: Radical prostatectomy and adjuvant endocrine treatment: a review. In: Schröder FH (ed) EORTC Genitourinary Group Monograph 8: Treatment of Prostatic Cancer: Facts and Controversies. Alan R Liss, New York 1990 (in press)

Surgical versus Medical Castration in the Management of Advanced Prostate Cancer

M.R.G. Robinson

Department of Urology, General Infirmary, Friarwood Lane, Pontefract, West Yorkshire WF8 1PL, United Kingdom

For centuries the effect of castration on sexuality and the secondary sex glands of man has been known and for the whole of this century orchidectomy has been employed as endocrine therapy for prostatic disorders. It was in 1786 that John Hunter first described scientifically the effect of castration on the prostate gland and at the end of the last century White [2] and Cabot [3] advocated, without distinguishing between benign and neoplastic disease, the removal of the testes for prostatic obstruction of the bladder neck. In 1941, Huggins et al. [4] stated that "in many instances, a malignant prostatic tumour is an overgrowth of adult prostatic epithelial cells. All known types of adult prostatic epithelial cells undergo atrophy when androgenic hormones are greatly reduced in amount. Therefore, significant improvement should occur in the clinical condition of patients with advanced prostatic carcinoma subjected to castration". The authors observed that, following orchidectomy, patients with advanced prostatic cancer experience relief of pain associated with calcification of lytic bone metastases and a fall in pre-treatment elevated acid phosphatase levels. They also observed that the administration of exogenous testosterone caused a return of symptoms. The only disadvantages of orchidectomy are the psychological stress of the operation, minor surgical complications such as scrotal haematoma or abscess, loss of libido and impotence, hot flushes and occasional transient ankle oedema. Since 1941, because of observations of Huggins, surgical castration has been the standard endocrine treatment against which other therapies have been judged. It was not until the early 1970s that plasma testosterone levels were first measured, demonstrating that castration does remove the principal source of androgens. It was observed that orchidectomy reduced the circulating plasma testosterone by 90% to castrate levels, with the remaining androgens being derived from the adrenal cortex [5,6]. Testosterone is a pro-hormone which is converted in the prostatic cell by 5-alpha reductase to dihydrotestosterone, the active hormone. The significance of dihydrotestosterone derived from adrenal androgens is discussed in other contributions to this monograph, but in spite of its existence it has generally been accepted that in symptomatic advanced prostatic carcinoma 70-80% of patients have a subjective or objective response to castration.

Clinical Studies; Orchidectomy

There have been few randomised prospective comparative studies of surgical castration versus other hormonal therapy in the treatment of prostatic cancer. Nesbitt and Baum [7], comparing patients treated by orchidectomy or oestrogen therapy with the historical controls described by Nesbit and Plum [8], claimed that in stage C of the disease there is an improvement in survival following both treatments. They were the first to observe that, when all cases of prostatic cancer are considered, the stage of the disease is of more prognostic significance than the treatment.

The first large randomised study was that of the Veterans Administrative Cooperative

Urological Research Group [9]. Patients with Veterans Stage C and D disease (locally advanced metastatic carcinoma of the prostate) were randomised to receive either placebo (in reality deferred treatment as all received therapy on progression), diethylstilboestrol 5 mg daily, orchidectomy and placebo, or orchidectomy and diethylstilboestrol. This study demonstrated that in Stage C of the disease, oestrogens given at this dosage may in fact have decreased survival because of the high incidence of cardiovascular disease, and that in Stage D disease, orchidectomy or any other treatment gives no benefit in terms of survival. More recently, a 3-armed EORTC randomised study, Protocol 30805 [10], comparing orchidectomy versus orchidectomy plus cyproterone acetate 50 mg 3 times a day versus diethylstilboestrol 1 mg daily, have shown no difference in time to progression and survival in patients with advanced metastatic prostatic carcinoma. The outcome in these patients has been shown to be determined by such prognostic factors as performance status, pain, histological differentiation of the primary tumour and alkaline phosphatase (not acid phosphatase) levels in the blood at the time of entry into the study. It can, therefore, be concluded that surgical castration results in excellent subjective response in terms of pain relief and improved performance status in the majority of patients with advanced prostatic carcinoma, with an objective measurable response in some patients. The outcome of the disease in terms of time to progression and survival is determined by the clinical stage of the disease and other prognostic factors.

Medical Castration

Many clinicians and some patients believe that, even though orchidectomy results in excellent palliation of symptoms in patients with advanced prostatic carcinoma, it is unacceptable for psychological reasons and because it is irreversible. Oestrogens which suppress circulating testosterone by blocking the feedback mechanisms involving luteinising hormone, as well as having a direct cytotoxic action on the prostatic cancer cells, were considered a suitable alternative to medical castration until the Veterans Cooperative Group's studies demonstrated their severe cardiovascular toxicity. Since their report of 1967 other alternatives have been sought. One of these is medical castration.

The stimulus for interstitial cells of the testis to produce testosterone is Luteinising Hormone (LH) from the anterior pituitary gland under the influence of Luteinising Hormone Releasing Hormone (LHRH) produced in the hypothalamus. LHRH was first isolated by Schally in 1961 and is a decapeptide [11]. Analogues of this hormone with a greatly increased activity compared to the natural hormone have since been developed. Paradoxically, when given in supraphysiological doses after the initial stimulation of LH, they inhibit its production, resulting in decreased testicular steroidogenesis. This is due to a loss or down-grading of gonadotrophin receptors in the hypothalamus. Some of these analogues, including buserelin, leuprolide and zoladex, are available for clinical use. They are not absorbed by mouth and have to be given transnasally by sniffing, or by injection. Long-term depot preparations of these substances are now available to be given by subcutaneous injection at monthly or longer intervals.

In 1983, Wenderoth and Jacobi [12], using buserelin acetate, demonstrated that there was an initial rise in serum testosterone during the first weeks of therapy. After approximately 21 days, testosterone fell to castrate levels. It is associated with a rise in plasma LH levels during the first weeks, following which they also fall to negligible levels. There have been reports that the initial rise of plasma testosterone may be associated with an exacerbation or flare of symptoms. In a study of 158 patients receiving the depot zoladex preparation given by monthly injection, Denis et al. [13] reported a transient increase in bone pain in 6 patients with 1 patient developing ureteric obstruction and 1 paraplegia during the first month of treatment. All patients recovered and continued in the study after showing a partial remission at the 3-month evaluation. In this study, 53% of the patients achieved a partial objective response, 19% had stable disease and 28% demonstrated disease progression. These results are similar to those achieved by surgical castration. Bouffioux et al. [14] reported that the flare of disease symptoms occurs in about 5-10% of patients with metastatic prostatic cancer who are treated with LHRH analogues alone. This may be prevented by giving an anti-androgen or diethylstilboestrol during the first 2 to 4 weeks of LHRH analogue therapy.

In addition to the initial flare of symptoms that is occasionally associated with LHRH analogues, the side effects are very similar to those of surgical orchidectomy. They include impotency and loss of libido together with hot flushes. The largest clinical trial comparing surgical and medical castration was undertaken by several centres in the United Kingdom and has been reported by Peeling [15]. Patients with advanced metastatic carcinoma of the prostate were randomised to be given zoladex or have a total or subcapsular orchidectomy. Three hundred and fifty-eight patients were entered into this study, of whom 182 were randomised to receive zoladex and 176 to undergo orchidectomy. In the early days of the trial, 36 of the patients receiving zoladex had the drug delivered by daily injections. Subsequently, the depot zoladex preparation became available and all patients were treated by monthly injections of this preparation. Of the total number of patients entered, 292 were fully evaluable. No significant differences were found between the subjective and objective responses that were observed in the 2 treatment arms. A few patients receiving zoladex experienced a mild increase in bone pain during the first few days of treatment. There were no cases of ureteric obstruction. One patient in each treatment arm developed paraplegia within the first month of treatment. It can be concluded, therefore, that the flare phenomenon is not a major clinical problem, even when medical castration with an LHRH analogue is not combined with an anti-androgen or oestrogen during the first few weeks of treatment.

In 1982, Labrie [16] introduced the concept of total androgen blockade. He suggested that either medical or surgical castration would be combined with the administration of pure anti-androgens, such as flutamide, to obtain the most effective treatment for prostatic cancer. The addition of such non-steroidal anti-androgen blocks the uptake of that DHT which is formed from adrenal androgens by the cell nucleus. It has been observed that, when flutamide is given alone, there is a secondary rise of testosterone during the first weeks of treatment. Theoretically, this overwhelms the action of the anti-androgen at the cellular level. Several studies of medical or surgical castration alone versus medical or surgical castration plus pure anti-androgen are in progress. The study of Crawford [17] suggests combination therapy is significantly beneficial in terms of progression and survival. This has not yet been confirmed by ongoing studies being undertaken by the Danish Prostatic Cancer Research Group or EORTC GU Group (personal communication).

Conclusion

In terms of time to progression, survival, subjective and objective response, there is no significant clinical difference between surgical and medical castration. Medical castration can produce a flare of symptoms in a small number of patients. This can be overcome by administering oestrogen or anti-androgens during the first few weeks of therapy. Castration may be unacceptable psychologically to some patients, but otherwise the side effects of both methods of castration are similar. Because medical castration is reversible, it may in the future find a role in determining those patients who are hormone dependent before they are subjected to irreversible surgical castration or treated by cytotoxic chemotherapy. Surgical castration has a great advantage over medical castration in that it is far less costly.

REFERENCES

1 Hunter J: Observation on Certain Parts of the Animal Oeconomy. First Edition, London 1786 p 39

2 White JW: Results of double castration in hypertrophy of the prostate. Ann Surg 1895 (22):1

3 Cabot AT: A question of castration for enlarged prostate. Ann Surg 1896 (24):265

4 Huggins C, Stevens RA, Hodges CB: Studies on prostatic cancer. II. The effects of castration on advanced carcinoma of the prostate gland. Arch Surg 1941 (43):209

5 Robinson MRG, Thomas BS: Effect of hormonal therapy on plasma testosterone levels in prostatic carcinoma. Br Med J 1971 (5):391-394

6 Shearer RJ, Hendry WF, Sommerville F, Fergusson JD: Plasma testosterone: an accurate monitor of hormone treatment in prostatic cancer. Br J Urol 1973 (45):468-477

7 Nesbitt RM, Baum WC: Endocrine control of prostatic carcinoma: clinical statistical survey of 1818 cases. JAMA 1950 (143):1317-1320

8 Nesbitt RM, Plumb RT: Prostatic carcinoma: a follow-up of 795 patients treated prior to endocrine era and a comparison of survival rates between these patients treated by endocrine therapy. Surgery 1946 (20):263-272

9 Veterans Administration Cooperative Urological Research Group: Treatment survival of patients with cancer of the prostate. Surg Gyn Obst 1967 (124):1011-1017

10 Robinson MRG: EORTC protocol 30805: a phase III trial comparing orchidectomy versus orchidectomy and cyproterone acetate and low dose stilboestrol in the management of metastatic carcinoma of the prostate. Smith PH, Pavone-Macaluso M (eds) Management of Advanced Cancer of the Prostate and Bladder. A Liss, New York 1988 pp 101-110

11 Schally AV, Arimura A, Baba Y, Mair RMG, Matsuo H, Redding TW, Debeljuk L: Isolation of properties of the FSH and LH releasing hormone. Biochem Biophys Res Comm 1971 (43):393-399

12 Wenderoth UK, Jacobi GH: Gonadotrophin-releasing hormone analogues in the palliation of carcinoma of the prostate. World J Urol 1983 (1):40

13 Denis L, Kuyppens F, Mahler C, Debruyne FMJ, Weil EHJ, Lunglmayr G, Newling D, Robinson MRG, Richards B, Smith PH, Whelan P: Long-term therapy with depot LHRH analogue (zoladex) in patients with advanced prostatic cancer. In: Murphy GP, Khoury S, Kuss R, Chatelane Ch and Denis L (eds) The Prostate Cancer. Part A: Research, Endocrine Treatment, Histopathology. A Liss, New York 1987 pp 221-228

14 Bouffioux C, Denis L, Mahler C, de Laval J: The treatment of advanced prostatic cancer with LHRH analogues: prevention of "flare-up" phenomenon. In: Murphy GP, Khoury S, Kuss R, Chatelane Ch and Denis L (eds) The Prostate Cancer. Part A: Research, Endocrine Treatment, Histopathology. A Liss, New York 1987 pp 255-260

15 Peeling WB: A comparison between surgical orchidectomy and LHRH antagonist ("Zoladex" ICI 188630). In: Murphy GP, Khoury S (eds) The Treatment of Metastatic Cancer of the Prostate. Therapeutic Progress in Urological Cancers. A Liss, New York 1989 pp 41-46

16 Labrie F, Dupont A, Belanger A, Cusan L, Lacousiere Y, Monfette G, Laberge JG, Emond JP, Fazekas ATA, Raynaud JP, Husson JM: New hormonal therapy in prostatic carcinoma: combined treatment with LHRH agonist and an anti-androgen. J Clin Invest Med 1982 (5):267-275

17 Crawford ED, Eisenberger MA, McLeod DJ, Spaulding JT, Benson R, Dorr FA, Blumenstral, Davis MA, Goodan DJ: A controlled trial of luprolide and flutamide in prostatic carcinoma. N Engl J Med 1989 (321):419-424

Second-Line Endocrine Treatment in Advanced Prostate Cancer

C. Mahler

Department of Endocrinology, Algemeen Ziekenhuis Middelheim, Lindendreef 1, 2020 Antwerp, Belgium

Primary failure of first-line endocrine therapy is seen in about 20% of all prostatic cancers and is attributed to hormonal independence or to unresponsiveness of the tumour. Secondary failure occurs when an initially responsive cancer escapes the control of the first-line endocrine treatment (orchidectomy, oestrogens, LHRH analogues, antiandrogens), the testosterone levels still being under castration values. This escape is considered to be due to the selection and/or cloning of pre-existing or *de novo* appearing hormone-resistant cell lines and occurs in the majority of patients within a period of 18 to 30 months after the start of treatment.

If one accepts the concept of hormonal resistance, then there is no good rationale to initiate secondary hormonal manipulation. Nevertheless, it has been shown that the administration of testosterone to these patients induces an immediate aggravation of the tumoural proces. On the other hand, as all clinicians know, there will be a response in about 30% of all patients when second-line endocrine treatment is started. This response, however, which is rarely objective, seldom exceeds a mean period of 6 months, following which the disease will progress. These observations imply that some hormone sensitivity remains, even after failure of initial therapy.

At present there is no clear-cut, well-established rule for second-line endocrine management. The varying sets of criteria used by different investigators to evaluate responses, make comparisons of different therapeutic regimens very difficult. In this chapter, we will discuss the currently available options for second-line endocrine therapy in progressive prostatic cancer, and their rationale.

Orchidectomy

Orchidectomy can be considered as second-line therapy when the initial medical treatment fails to achieve a satisfactory reduction of plasma testosterone [1].

Many urologists feel that orchidectomy should be performed in all patients after failure of primary treatment and before a new hormonal therapy is started. This makes good sense since, following the cessation of initial medical therapy, testosterone levels might rise again and enhance tumour growth. There is ample clinical evidence that, after castration, at least some cancer cells remain hormone sensitive, as has been shown by the fact that 40% to 50% of patients in relapse will somehow respond to antiandrogens and/or medical or surgical adrenal castration [2-5]. Review of the literature yields few reports on the effects of orchidectomy as second-line therapy [6-12]. Overall response was nearly 20%, but rarely lasted more than 6 months.

Oestrogens

Due to the severe and sometimes lethal side effects and complications of oestrogens, many authors feel that these substances should no longer be used in the management of advanced prostatic cancer, although the VACURG studies reported less cancer-related deaths. Recent reports are quite scarce. There is a low incidence and brief duration of objective responses [12]. There is some renewed interest in the administration of high

Table 1. Comparison of reported results after bilateral adrenalectomy in advanced prostatic cancer [15-23]

Authors		N° patients	Obj.Res.	Subj.Res.	Duration (months)
Huggins	1945	4	-	3	4
Baker	1953	10	-	8	1-6
Scardino	1953	3	1	3	3-9
Whitmore	1954	17	2	11	11
Ferguson	1954	17	-	12	10
Morales	1955	20	1	9	3-24
McFarlane	1960	13	-	9	2-46
Schoonees	1972	13	11(?)	11	1-3
Mahoney	1972	22	1	18	?
Bhanalagh	1974	26	1	16	3-16

doses of diethylstilboestrol-diphosphate (fosfoestrol) and an ongoing study is currently evaluating the possible role of this compound.

Progestins and Progestational Antiandrogens

Progesterone compounds (hydroxy-progesterone caproate, chlormadinone acetate, megoestrol acetate and medroxyprogesterone acetate) have been widely used in secondary treatment of prostatic cancer, but the results have been very disappointing. Fossa et al., comparing medroxyprogesterone acetate (MPA) to prednisolone in relapsing patients, reported a superior response to MPA [13]. However, some of these substances might have androgenic properties and induce more harm than benefit to the patient.

Surgical Adrenalectomy

In 1945, Huggins and Scott performed bilateral adrenalectomy in patients with prostatic cancer in progression after castration, with the aim of further reducing circulating androgen levels [14]. Until the early seventies, adrenalectomy was an established procedure for relapsing patients. Table 1 reviews the main reported series of results in the literature. Objective responses are very rare, but subjective responses were noted in up to 70% of cases. When present, responses were short-lived and rarely lasted more than 6 months. Some authors attributed the temporary amelioration to the analgesic and euphoric effects of concomitant corticotherapy [24].

The high morbidity and mortality associated with this ablative procedure, together with the availability of new drugs able to induce medical adrenal suppression, have led to the abandonment of this type of surgical intervention.

Hypophysectomy

Hypophysectomy, either by surgical means or by irradiation, has mainly a pain-relieving effect. It is, except in a few institutions, no longer used in the management of relapsed patients [25].

Medical Adrenal Suppression

Several drugs are available today to suppress adrenal steroidogenesis in a reversible manner, and some of them have been used in the management of progressive prostatic cancer.

Table 2. Responses reported in the management of progressive prostatic cancer in relapse with a combination of AG and hydrocortisone [27-35]

Authors		N° patients	Obj.Res. %	Subj.Res. %	St.Dis. %	Progression %
Robinson	1974	26	0	5	-	-
Rostom	1982	15	0	0	41	59
Lippman	1983	12	0	0	40	60
Bauer	1984	10	0	0	30	-
Block	1984	23	0	0	0	100
Drago	1984	35	3	17	29	51
Murray	1987	126	17	-	22	61
Crawford	1987	129	0	10	39	50
Elomaa	1988	20	20	75	-	

Aminoglutethimide (AG)

AG, which was initially used as an anticonvulsive agent, blocks the transformation of cholesterol to pregnenolone, a precursor of the corticosteroids. It is also an effective aromatase inhibitor. Used as monotherapy and depending on the dose, it can completely suppress adrenal function, requiring substitutive doses of cortisone to prevent Addisonian crises [26]. Table 2 evaluates some of the effects of AG reported in the literature.

From this comparison it appears that, even if no identical response criteria are used, this combined therapy might be of benefit to a small minority of patients. The amelioration is mainly subjective, with improved performance status and decrease of pain. Improved survival time is reported by Murray. Side effects are dose dependent (500 to 1000 mg/day): lethargy, lassitude, gastro-intestinal complaints and orthostatic hypotension have been reported. Dose reduction or withdrawal is sometimes necessary. Perry et al., comparing AG to physiological doses of hydrocortisone alone, question the therapeutic efficacy of AG and conclude that hydrocortisone induces superior results [36]. Labrie et al. combine AG with antiandrogens in relapsing patients and claim some objective response with this regimen [37].

Trilostane

Trilostane inhibits 3-hydroxysteroid dehydrogenase and has been used in treating Cushing and Conn syndromes. Trials to evaluate its role in the manipulation of prostatic cancer are limited [38].

Ketoconazole

Ketoconazole is a derivative of the imidazole group, and is known as a broad-spectrum antimycotic agent. By interfering with the P 450 cytochrome complexes responsible for steroidogenesis, it blocks gonadal and adrenal androgen synthesis. This effect is dose dependent and entirely reversible upon cessation of treatment [39-41]. This potential has been exploited by several groups of investigators who used the drug in both first- and second-line endocrine therapy of prostatic cancer following Trachtenberg's first publication of positive responses to Ketoconazole [42]. The same author also reported a direct antitumour effect on prostatic cancer cells *in vitro* [43]. Table 3 summarises the responses seen in the principal reported series.

These data are comparable to our own experience with Ketoconazole. We did not see any objective response (EORTC criteria) but 8 out of 20 patients had subjective improvement for a mean period of 5 months (range 3-16 months) [53]. Secondary effects were frequent. Gastro-intestinal intolerance with nausea and vomiting (40%), fatigue, dryness of the skin and pruritus, nail dystrophy and abnormal liver function tests have been noted. Pain relief, however, is often impressive and although the side effects limit the use of this drug, it might be helpful in selected patients. As shown in Fig. 1, however, its interference

Table 3. Responses to Ketoconazole (high dose) in relapsing prostatic cancer [44-52]

		N° patients	Obj.Res.	Subj.Res.	St. Dis.	Duration (months)
Debruyne	1986	39	0	21	23	-
Williams	1986	20	1	11	2	-
Bredt	1986	15	8	3	-	1-12
Van Cangh	1986	14	0	4	4	3-9
Pont	1987	11	0	5	4	-
Havlin	1987	15	0	3	6	3-4
MacKintosh	1987	12	0	0	10	-
Johnson	1988	22	2	13	7	3-8
Jubelirer	1989	16	0	2	6	3-12

with adrenal steroidogenesis implies the risk of adrenal insufficiency and this requires regular monitoring of cortisol levels.

R.75251

R.75251 is a new imidazole derivative with increased potency , as compared to Ketoconazole. Through interaction with cytochrome P-450-dependent enzymes, it strongly inhibits testicular androgen synthesis in healthy male volunteers. In a pilot study on 24 orchidectomised and relapsed prostate cancer patients, a 300 mg b.i.d. dose regimen

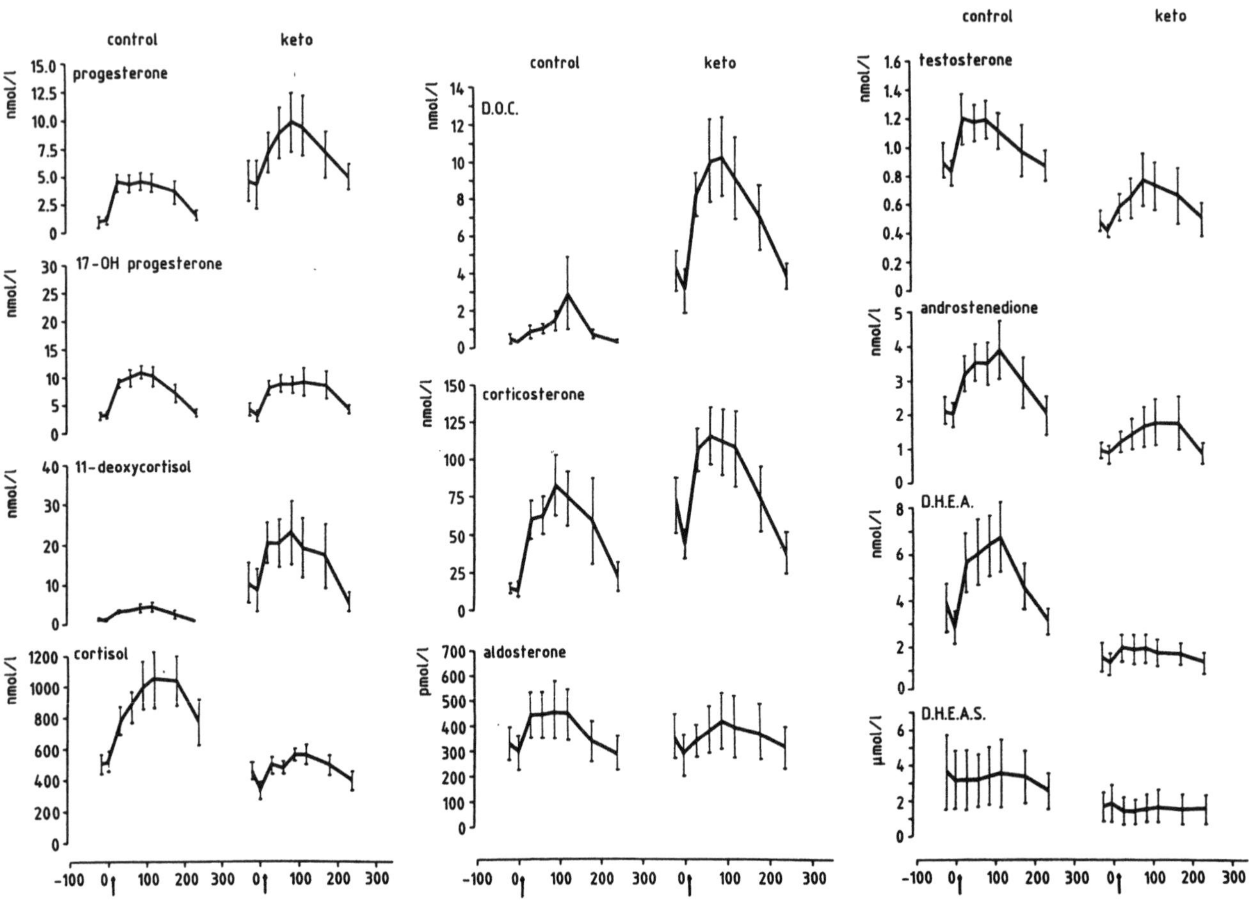

Fig. 1. Adrenal hormonal responses to an acute ACTH challenge before (control) and during Ketokonazole therapy

had positive effects on bone pain, urological complaints and tumour volume, with decrease of PSA values. We were able to show that the mecanisms of action of this compound are not mediated by its interference with adrenal androgens [54]. Studies to elucidate the pathways of its antitumoural effect are currently in progress and there is already some evidence that raised tissue levels of retinoic acid might be one of the mechanisms involved. Side effects mainly affected the skin and nails. Gastro-intestinal tolerance was good.

Antiandrogens

Antiandrogens, either steroidal (cyproterone acetate; CPA) or non-steroidal (flutamide, anandron or casodex) are increasingly being used as a first-line modality in monotherapy or combined treatment, in order to induce complete androgen blockade [55]. In relapsing patients, these drugs can be used to evaluate their blocking effect on adrenal androgens. In most cases, responses are rare and short-lived [56-64]. Although these substances are generally well tolerated, they can, in some patients, cause severe side effects (gastro-intestinal intolerance, hepatotoxicity) [64-65].

Other Hormones or Drugs with Hormonal Effects

Calcitonin, spironolactone and diphosphonates have been used as therapeutic adjuvants in the management of progressive prostatic cancer. Responses are minimal. Some beneficial action has been reported with Tamoxifen, an antioestrogen [66]. Priming of cancer cells with androgens before administration of cytotoxic chemotherapy did not improve the efficacy of this therapeutic modality [67].

Another hormone is at present being investigated for its potential effects in cancer therapy. Somatostatine (SMS) and its more potent analogues are known inhibitors of different hormonal systems. As far as prostatic cancer is concerned, we know that SMS blocks GH, PRL and tissular growth factors. A direct antiproliferative effect has been shown. Schally and coworkers reported the inhibitory effects of an SMS analogue, given alone or in association with an LHRH analogue, on tumour growth in the Dunning R 3327 prostate cancer model [68]. Bogden et al. used the BIM 23014 analogue and also showed significant results. It is noteworthy that, even in some non-hormone-dependent cancer strains of the prostate, a similar inhibitory effect was observed [69]. We have started a trial with such an analogue (Sandostatine ®) in patients in relapse.

Estramustine (Estracyt ®)

Two other hormones, oestradiol and prednisone (bound to nitrogen mustard, an alkylating agent), might have simultaneous hormonal and cytotoxic effects. The first and best known agent is estramustine phosphate (nor-nitrogen mustard + oestradiol-17-phosphate). It has been extensively used in first- and second-line management of prostatic cancer. The rationale is to carry the drug to the prostatic cell through a receptor binding to a specific protein that has been shown to be present in the prostate. Its effects are thought to be simultaneously cytotoxic and oestrogenic. The cytotoxic impact of Estracyt is mediated through its interaction with the cellular microtubular complex. Estramustine has been evaluated in many phase II and several randomised phase III trials in patients who had become refractory to conventional therapy. The reported results are conflicting but this drug is, nevertheless, considered to be a valuable alternative in relapsing patients, with an overall response rate of 30% to 35%. Side effects (similar to those of oestrogens) are common and can be expected in about 10% of patients. A more extensive review of this medication is found in an article by I. Könyves [70]. A second compound, Prednimustine, is still being investigated.

Suramin

Very recently, a "new" old drug, Suramin, has stirred considerable interest. Suramin is a polysulphonated naphtylurea that has been used in the treatment of Rhodesian and Gambian trypanosomiasis and onchocercosis since the early 1920s. It is a potent reverse transcriptase inhibitor and has exhibited some anti-HIV activity *in vitro*. It has also been shown to block the binding of several types of growth factors, including platelet-derived growth factor (PDGF), transforming growth factor-beta (TGF-B) and epidermal growth factor (EGF), to their corresponding cell surface receptors, and preliminary reports have documented objective responses in tumour cells in tissue culture. Winnann et al. reported its activity in relapsing prostatic cancer, where especially patients with extensive local and lymph-nodal tumour burden or with low-volume bone metastases seemed to respond with relief of pain and a decrease in PSA values (7 out of 11 patients) [71]. Our own, as yet unpublished data, yield evidence of some partial response.

However, this drug has serious side effects and severe toxicity. Often, fever up to 40° C is seen during or immediately after intravenous administration. Nausea, malaise, rash and myalgia are frequent. Neurological dysfunctions: paraesthesia, peripheral neuropathy and even the Guillain Barré syndrome, can occur. Adrenal insufficiency, hepatotoxicity and coagulation disorders have been noted. For these reasons, strict monitoring of plasma suramin levels and a close follow-up of the patient are absolutely mandatory.

Conclusions

Treatment of patients with progressive prostatic cancer after failure of first-line endocrine therapy remains disappointing for physicians and patients alike. Whatever second-line endocrine regimen is chosen, the response is often similar. At best there is some subjective improvement lasting for approx. 6 months, but most patients will have died within one year. This explains why some authors feel that second-line therapy in failing patients should only be initiated when the patients have become truly symptomatic.

As long as we are unable to offer better curative prospects, we should look for the most acceptable and affordable palliative treatment, taking into account the patient's specific wishes. Quality of survival is more important than length of survival. Table 4 recapitulates the main therapeutic modalities, their contraindications, side effects and administration regimens.

Acknowledgement

I am indebted to Prof. Dr. L. Denis for his help and collaboration and to Mrs. G. Clever for her skillful secretarial assistance.

Table 4. Practical information about the main therapeutic modalities in second-line endocrine treatment

Orchidectomy:	total or subcapsular	
Oestrogens:	contraindications:	cardiovascular disease
	side effects:	cardiovascular complications
		thrombo-embolic disease
		hypertension
		salt and fluid retention
		gynaecomastia
	most used drug:	diethylstilboestrol 3 mg/day
		stilboestrol diphosphate per os and i.v.
	proprietary name:	Honvan

Table 4. Practical information about the main therapeutic modalities in second-line endocrine treatment (continued)

Progestins:	contraindications:	cardiovascular disease diabetes
	side effects:	gastro-intestinal dysfunction fluid retention gynaecomastia altered liver function tests
	most used drug:	medroxyprogesterone acetate
	proprietary name:	Farlutal per os and i.v.
Aminoglutethimide:	contraindications:	intolerance
	side effects:	lethargy, somnolence gastro-intestinal dysfunction orthostatic hypotension adrenal insufficiency
	proprietary name:	Orimeten 125 and 250 mg b.i.d. or t.i.d.
	should be given with hydrocortisone 30 mg/day	
Ketoconazole:	contraindication:	acute hepatic disease
	side effects:	gastro-intestinal intolerance dry skin, pruritus, nail dystrophy gynaecomastia adrenal insufficiency
	proprietary name:	Nizoral 600 to 1200 mg/day
R.75251:	still under investigation	
Cyproterone acetate:	contraindications:	acute hepatic disease thrombo-embolic disease diabetes
	side effects:	gynaecomastia cardio-vascular complications altered hepatic function tests fatigue
	proprietary names:	Androcur 300 mg/day Cyprostat
Flutamide:	contraindications:	as for CPA
	side effects:	similar to those of CPA
	proprietary name:	Eulexin 250 mg t.i.d.
Nilutamide:	contraindications:	as for CPA
	side effects:	idem blurred vision
	proprietary name:	Anandron100 mg t.i.d.
Tamoxifen:	side effects:	hot flushes, fatigue gastro-intestinal dysfunction dry skin, blurred vision
	proprietary name:	Nolvadex 20 to 40 mg/day
Estramustine phosphate:	contraindications:	as for oestrogens
	side effects:	as for oestrogens
	proprietary name:	Estracyt 450 to 750 mg/day i.m.
Prednimustine:	still under investigation	
Suramin:	contraindications:	renal diseases, coagulopathy
	side effects:	immediate reaction: nausea, rash, fever, shock hepatic toxicity, albuminuria, paraesthesia adrenal insufficiency
	proprietary names:	Germanin, Moranyl
	should only be given under close monitoring of suramin levels	

REFERENCES

1 Nesbit RM and Baum WC: Endocrine control of prostatic carcinoma. Clinical and statistical survey of 1,818 cases. JAMA 1950 (143):1317-1320

2 Robinson RMG, Shearer RJ, Fergusson JD: Adrenal suppression in the treatment of carcinoma of the prostate. Br J Urol 1974 (46):555

3 Stoliar B, Albert DJ: SCH 13521 in the treatment of advanced carcinoma of the prostate. J Urol 1974 (111):803

4 Sogani PC, Ray B, Whitmore WF Jr: Advanced prostatic carcinoma: flutamide therapy after conventional endocrine treatment. Urology 1975 (6):164

5 Labrie F, Dupont A, Bélanger A, Giguère M, Borsanyi JP, Lacourcière Y, Emond J, Monfette G, Lachance R: The importance of combination therapy with Flutamide and castration (LHRH agonist or orchiectomy) in previously untreated as well as previously treated patients with advanced prostate cancer. In: JGM Klijn, R Paridaens, JA Foekens (eds) Hormonal Manipulation of Cancer: Peptides, Growth Factors and (Anti)-Steroidal Agents. Raven Press, New York 1986

6 Jordan WP, Blackard CE and Byar DP: Reconsideration of orchiectomy in the treatment of advanced prostatic carcinoma. South Med J 1977 (70):1411-1413

7 Biorn CL, Gray CP and Strauss E: Orchiectomy after presumed estrogen failure in treatment of carcinoma of the prostate. West J Med 1979 (130):363-364

8 Frenster JH, Hovsepian JA and the VACURG Group: Regained response to stilbestrol therapy after orchiectomy in advanced prostate carcinoma. Proc Amer Ass Cancer Res 1979 (20):296

9 Stone AR, Hargreave TB and Chisholm GD: The diagnosis of oestrogen escape and the role of secondary orchiectomy in prostatic cancer. Br J Urol 1980 (52):535-538

10 Denis L and Nowé P: Bilateral orchiectomy in patients with progressive advanced prostatic cancer. Acta Urol Belg 1980 (48):113-116

11 Klugo RC, Farah RN and Cerny JC: Bilateral orchiectomy for carcinoma of prostate. Urology 1981 (17):49-50

12 Klijn JGM, Nielander AJM, Alexieva-Figusch J, Van Putten WLJ: Orchidectomy and oestrogens as secondary forms of treatment for metastatic prostatic cancer. In: Schroeder FH, Richards B (eds) Therapeutic Principles in Metastatic Prostatic Cancer. Alan R Liss, New York 1985 pp 335-349

13 Fossa SD, Ogreid P, Karlsen S, Havelan H, Jensen J, Trovag A: High dose medroxyprogesterone acetate (MPA) versus prednisolone (P) in hormone-resistant prostatic cancer. In: Bracci U, Di Silverio F (eds) Advances in Urological Oncology and Endocrinology. Acta Medica, Rome1984 pp 433-437

14 Huggins C, Scott W: Bilateral surrenalectomy in prostatic cancer. Ann Surg 1945 (122):1031

15 Baker WJ: Bilateral adrenalectomy for carcinoma of the prostate gland. Preliminary Report. J Urol 1953 (70/2):275

16 Scardino PL, Prince CL, McGoldrick TA: Bilateral adrenalectomy for prostatic cancer. J Urol 1953 (70/1):100

17 Whitmore WF, Randall HT, Pearson OH, West CD: Adrenalectomy in the treatment of prostatic cancer. Geriatrics 1954 (9):62

18 Fergusson JD: Total adrenalectomy for malignant disease of the prostate and breast. Proc Royal Soc Med 1954 (47):1007

19 Morales PA, Brendler H, Hotchkiss RS: The role of the adrenal cortex in prostatic cancer. J Urol 195 (73/2):399

20 Mac Farlane DA, Thomas LP, Harrison JH: A survey of total adrenalectomy in cancer of the prostate. Am J Surg 1960 (99):562

21 Schoonees R, Schalch DC, Reynoso G, Murphy GP: Bilateral adrenalectomy for advanced prostatic carcinoma. J Urol 1972 (108/1):123

22 Mahoney EM, Harrison JH: Bilateral adrenalectomy for palliative treatment of prostatic cancer. J Urol 1972 (108):936

23 Bhanalaph T, Varkarakis M, Murphy G: Current status of bilateral adrenalectomy on advanced prostatic carcinoma. Ann Surg 1974 (179):17-23

24 Miller G, Hinnan F: Cortisone treatment in advanced carcinoma of the prostate. J Urol (Baltimore)1954 (72):486-496

25 Fergusson JD: Limits and indications for adrenalectomy and hypophysectomy in the treatment of prostatic cancer. In: Bracci, Di Silverio (eds) Hormonal Therapy of Prostatic Cancer. Cofese Edizioni, Palermo 1975 pp 201-207

26 Sanford E, Drago J, Rohner T et al: Aminoglutethimide medical adrenalectomy for advanced prostatic cancer. J Urol (Baltimore) 1976 (115):170-174

27 Robinson MRG, Shearer RJ, Fergusson JD: Adrenal suppression in the treatment of carcinoma of the prostate. Br J Urol1974 (46):444-559

28 Rostom AY, Folkes A, Lord C, Notley RG, Schweitzer FAW and White WF: Aminoglutethimide therapy for advanced carcinoma of the prostate. Br J Urol 1982 (54):552-555

29 Lippman A et al: Aminoglutethimide for metastatic prostatic cancer. Proc ASCO 1983 (144) abstr C-563

30 Bauer HW, Schmeller NT, Schmiedt E: Adrenal suppression with aminoglutethimide in advanced prostatic carcinoma. J Urol 1984 (131):207A (abstr 413)

31 Block M, Trump D, Rose DP, Cummings KB, Hogan TF: Evaluation of aminoglutethimide in stage D prostate cancer: an assessment of efficacy and toxicity in patients with tumors refractory to hormonal therapy. Cancer Treat Rep 1984 (68):719-722.

32 Drago JR, Santen RJ, Lipton A, Worgul TJ, Harvey HA, Boucher A, Manni A, Rohner TJ: Clinical effect of aminoglutethimide, medical adrenalectomy, in treatment of 43 patients with advanced prostatic carcinoma. Cancer 1984 (53):1447-1450

33 Murray R, Pitt P: Aminoglutethimide in the treatment of advanced prostatic cancer. In: Murphy GP, Khoury S, Kuss R, Chatelain C, Denis L (eds) Prostate Cancer. Part A: Research, Endocrine

Treatment and Histopathology. Alan R Liss, New York 1987 pp 275-282
34 Crawford ED, Ahmann FR, Davis MA, Levasseur YJ: Aminoglutethimide in metastatic adenocarcinoma of the prostate. In: Murphy GP, Khoury S, Kuss R, Chatelain C, Denis L (eds): Prostate Cancer. Part A: Research, Endocrine Treatment and Histopathology. Alan R Liss, New York 1987 pp 283-289
35 Elomaa I, Taube T, Blomqvist C, Rissanen P, Rannikko S, Alfthan O: Amino-glutethimide for advanced prostatic cancer resistant to conventional hormonal therapy. Eur Urol 1988 (14):104-106
36 Perry LA, Plowman PN, Rowell NP, Chard T: Androgen suppression by hydrocortisone without aminoglutethimide in orchidectomised men with prostate cancer. In: Abstract Book International Symposium on Hormonal Manipulation of Cancer: Peptides, Growth Factors and New (Anti)steroidal Agents. Rotterdam, June 4-6 1986 p 110
37 Labrie F, Dupont A, Giguère M, Borsanyi JP, Lacourcière Y, Bélanger A, Lachance R, Emond J, Monfette G: Combination therapy with flutamide and castration (orchidectomy or LHRH agonist): the minimal endocrine therapy in both untreated and previously treated patients with advanced cancer of the prostate and bladder.In: Smith PH, Pavone-Macaluso M (eds) Management of Advanced Cancer of the Prostate and Bladder. Alan R Liss, New York 1988 pp 41-62
38 Beardwell CG: Clinical use of trilostane. In: Furr BSA and Wakeling AE (eds) Pharmacology and Clinical Uses of Inhibitors of Hormone Secretion and Action. Baillière Tindall, London 1986
39 Van den Bossche H, Lauwers W, Willemsens G, Cools W: Ketoconazole, an inhibitor of the cytochrome P-450-dependent testosterone synthesis. In: Schroeder FH, Richards B (eds) EORTC Genito-Urinary Group, Monograph 2, Part A: Therapeutic Principles in Metastatic Prostatic Cancer. Alan R Liss, New York 1985 pp 187-196
40 Pont A, Williams PL, Azhar S, Reitz RE, Bochra CH, Smith ER, Stevens DA: Ketoconazole blocks testosterone synthesis.Arch Intern Med 1982 (142):2137-2140
41 Mahler C, Denis L, De Coster R: The endocrine effect of ketoconazole high doses (KHD). In: Murphy GP, Khoury S, Kuss R, Chatelain C, Denis L (eds) Prostate Cancer. Part A: Research, Endocrine Treatment and Histopathology. Alan R Liss, New York 1987 pp 291-297
42 Trachtenberg J, Halpern N and Pont A: Ketoconazole: a novel and rapid treatment for advanced prostatic cancer. J Urol 1987 (130 part 2):152
43 Trachtenberg J and Eichenberger T: Extra-hormonal effects of imidazoles on human prostatic cancer. J Urol 1987 (137 part 2):115A, abstract 45
44 Debruyne FMJ, Witjes J and Members of the Dutch South-East Cooperative Study Group: Ketoconazole high dose (HD) in the management of metastatic prostatic carcinoma. J Urol 1986 (135part 2):203A, abstract 397
45 Williams G, Kerle DJ, Ware H, Dobie A, Dunlop H, Smith C, Allen J, Yeo T and Bloom SR: Objective responses to ketoconazole therapy in patients with relapsed progressive prostatic cancer. Br J Urol 1986 (58):45
46 Bredt A, Brughers A, Girey G, Schottinger J, Helman N and Weisz J: Ketoconazole therapy for metastatic prostate cancer resistant to prior hormonal treatment. Proc Amer Soc Clin Oncol 1986 (5):99, abstract 385
47 Van Cangh PJ and Opsomer RJ: High dose ketoconazole as secondary form of therapy in metastatic prostatic cancer. J Urol 1986 (135 part 2):338A, abstract 934
48 Pont A: Long-term experience with high dose ketoconazole therapy in patients with stage D2 prostatic carcinoma. J Urol 1987 (137):902
49 Havlin K, Jordan VC, Cummings K, Messing E and Trump DL: Ketoconazole (KC) in advanced prostatic cancer (CaP) refractory to initial hormonal therapy: a clinical and endocrinologic study. Proc Amer Soc Clin Oncol 1987 (6):106 abstract 416
50 MacKintosh FR, Nickx CC, MacKintosh CL and Hall SW: High dose ketoconazole (K) therapy for metastatic prostatic cancer (MPC): a clinico-pharmacologic phase II study. Proc Amer Soc Clin 1987 (6):101 abstract 397
51 Johnson DE, Babaian RJ, von Eschenbach AC, Wishnow KI and Tenney D: Ketoconazole therapy for hormonally refractive metastatic prostate cancer. Urology 1988 (31):132
52 Jubelirer S and Hogan T: High dose ketoconazole for the treatment of hormone refractory metastatic prostatic carcinoma : 16 cases and review of the literature. J Urol 1989 (142):89-91
53 Mahler C: Ketoconazole. In: Khoury S and Chatelain C (eds) Urologie: Cancer de la Prostate. FIIS et RGP 1988 pp 365-368
54 Mahler C, Denis L and De Coster R: The effects of a new imidazole derivative in advanced prostatic cancer. A preliminary report. In: Murphy G and Khoury S (eds) Therapeutic Progress in Urological Cancers. Alan R Liss, New York 1989 pp 205-209
55 Labrie F, Dupont A, Bélanger A, Giguère M, Lacourcière Y, Emond J, Monfette G, Bergeron V: Combination therapy with Flutamide and castration (LHRH agonist or orchiectomy) in advanced prostate cancer: a marked improvement in response and survival. J Steroid Biochem 1985 (23):833
56 Bracci U, Di Silverio F: Terapia chirurgica ed ormonale del carcinoma prostatico. In: Bracci U, Di Silverio F (eds) Terapia dei tumori ormonodipendenti. Acta Medica, Rome 1979 pp 173-201
57 Giuliani L, Pescatore D, Giberti C, Martorana G, Natta G: Treatment of advanced prostatic carcinoma with cyproterone acetate and orchiectomy: 5 year follow-up. Eur Urol 1980 (6):145-148
58 Kaisary AV, Fellows GJ, Smith JC: Antiandrogen (flutamide) therapy in management of relapsing metastatic prostatic carcinoma. J Urol 1987 (137):256A
59 Di Silverio F, Tenaglia R, Bizzari M, Biggio A, Saragnano R: Experience with flutamide in advanced prostatic cancer patients refractory to previous endocrine therapy. J Drug Dev 1987(1 suppl 1):10-16

60 Habenicht UF, Schroeder H, El Etreby F, Neumann F: Advantages and disadvantages of pure antiandrogens and of antiandrogens of the cyproterone acetate-type in the treatment of prostatic cancer. In: Smith PH, Pavone-Macaluso M (eds): Management of Advanced Cancer of the Prostate and Bladder. Alan R Liss, New York 1988 pp 63-75
61 Beurton D, Grall J, Davody Ph and Cukier J: Treatment of prostatic cancer with cyproterone acetate as monotherapy. In: Murphy GP, Khoury S, Kuss R, Chatelain C, Denis L (eds) Prostate Cancer. Part A. Research, Endocrine Treatment and Histopathology. Alan R Liss, New York 1987 pp 369-378
62 Denis L: A new non-steroidal anti-androgen. In: Murphy G and Khoury S (eds) Therapeutic Progress in Urological Cancers. Alan R Liss, New York 1989 pp 205-209
63 Tunn UW: Cyproterone acetate in the management of prostatic cancer.In: Murphy G and Khoury S (eds) Therapeutic Progress in Urological Cancers. Alan R Liss, New York 1989 pp 205-209
64 Pavone-Macaluso M, Pavone C, Serreta V, Cacciatore M, Cavallo N, Romano C, Daricello G: Side-effects of various modalities of hormonal treatment of prostatic carcinoma. J Endocrinol Invest 1987 (10 suppl 2) abstract
65 MacFarlane JR, Tolley DA: Flutamide therapy for advanced prostatic cancer: a phase II study. Br J Urol 1985 (57):172-174
66 De Voogt HJ: Second-line endocrine management:anti androgens and anti-estrogens. In: Schroeder FH, Richards B (eds) Therapeutic Principles in Metastatic Prostate Cancer. Alan R Liss, New York 1985 pp 351-357
67 Manni A, Santen R, Boucher A, Lipton A, Harvey H, White D, Simmonds M, Gordon R, Rohner I, Drago J, Wettlaufer J, Glode L: Androgen priming and chemotherapy in advanced prostate cancer. J Endocrinol Invest 1987 (10 suppl 2):32
68 Schally AV, Redding TW: Somatostatin analogs as adjuncts to agonists of LHRH in the treatment of experimental prostate cancer. Proc Natl Acad Sci USA 1987 (84):7275-7279
69 Bogden A: Effects of BIM 23014 on prostatic tumours in the rat. In: BIM 23014. Information for Clinical Investigators. Ipsen Intern 1988
70 Könyves I: Estramustine Phosphate (Estracyt ®) in the treatment of prostatic carcinoma. Int Urol Nephrol 1989 (4):393-397
71 Winnan Ewing M, Larocca RV, Stein CA, Myers CE and Linehan WM: Effect of Suramin on proliferation of human prostate carcinoma. Proc Am Assoc Cancer Res 1989 (30):310

Chemotherapy for Advanced Prostate Cancer

Mario A. Eisenberger

Associate Professor of Medicine and Oncology, Department of Medicine and the University of Maryland Cancer Center, University of Maryland Medical Systems, 22 South Greene St., Baltimore, Maryland 21201, U.S.A.

The primary modality of treatment for patients with disseminated cancer of the prostate focusses on the suppression of androgenic stimulation of tumour growth. Androgen deprivation procedures of various kinds result in subjective/objective clinical benefits in the majority (70-80%) of patients with metastatic disease and, clearly, reflect some of the most effective systemic palliative treatments for solid tumours in man. Paradoxically however, the development of endocrine resistance, which is observed within a relatively predictable time frame, is an extraordinarily effective phenomenon. In prostate cancer, contrary to breast cancer, responses to second-line endocrine manipulations are uncommon, usually brief and subjective and, more important, have no impact on survival. Extensive data accumulated over the past few decades, derived from large-scale, prospective randomised trials testing various methods of androgen deprivation, have shown that the median time to progression and the median survival in cohorts of patients have consistently ranged from 12-18 months and 24-30 months, respectively [1,2]. These data also stress that the development of effective non-hormonal cytotoxic approaches is the key step in order to accomplish significant advances in the systemic treatment of this disease. Preclinical data have shown that various phenotypic changes are increasingly expressed in parallel with the development of endocrine resistance [3]. These may represent either somatic mutations from a hormonally sensitive to an insensitive state, expansion of previously insensitive cell clones, or, most likely, both [4].

Much effort is currently devoted to enhancing our understanding of the mechanisms involved in endocrine resistance and further knowledge in this field will undoubtedly allow clinicians to develop therapeutic approaches in a more rational and logical way. In the meantime, non-hormonal cytotoxic treatment for prostatic cancer has focussed on conventional chemotherapeutic agents, traditionally employed for the treatment of various human malignancies. The extensive data accumulated thus far is reviewed and summarised herein.

Evaluation of Therapeutic Efficacy

The difficulty in assessing response to treatment in this disease by using conventional criteria is a well recognised limitation. The application of the usual criteria for response employed in most clinical trials may only be possible in a smaller proportion of patients with evidence of bidimensionally measurable disease. The main problem is that metastatic cancer of the prostate most frequently manifests itself by osteoblastic bone lesions or mixed "blastic" and "lytic" lesions which are virtually impossible to quantitate prospectively in a reliable fashion. Evaluation of responses in bone metastasis are notoriously difficult to reproduce.

Table 1 illustrates the most commonly employed methods to evaluate the effects of chemotherapy (or other systemic treatments) in patients with metastatic disease. Probably no more than one-fourth of the patients with metastatic disease present with evidence of bidimensionally measurable disease, which allows investigators to quantitate certain disease sites along with treatment. Not uncom-

Table 1. Objective parameters most commonly used to assess responses in patients with endocrine-resistant prostatic cancer [1]

Method	Limitations
Bone radiographs	Lesions are predominantly blastic and usually will not change with treatment
Bone scans	Quantitative assessments of positive areas are difficult in both directions. More useful to document progression
Serum acid phosphatase[2]	Valuable only in rare occasions when very high values return to normal. Significant variations may be observed independent of treatment
Serum alkaline phosphatase	Usually do not correlate with response or progression after treatment
Measurement of prostatic size	Measurements are frequently unidimensional (digital exam). The use of transrectal ultrasound and prostatic CAT scan or magnetic resonance imaging are still controversial for monitoring response to treatment

1. Table modified from Eisenberger M, Kennedy P, Abrams J: Oncology 1987 1(4):59-69
2. Data with prostate-specific antigen (PSA) is still lacking at this time (1989)

monly, some patients demonstrate evidence of "mixed responses", i.e., improvement of soft tissue disease sites but increase or persistent symptomatology in other areas, most commonly bones. Patients with evidence of visceral organ involvement are frequently debilitated, have far advanced disease with extensive bone involvement and many times have received significant prior palliative radiotherapy, all of which usually limit optimal use of cytotoxic drugs. Similarly, the issue of whether patients with visceral involvement represent a subset of patients with different prognosis from those with bone disease only, remains unclear. While on the one hand the subset of patients with measurable disease may be more appropriate for clinical trials, it is possible that they also represent a subgroup that is less likely to respond to any treatment.

For several years, the National Prostatic Cancer Project (NPCP) has utilised criteria for response developed by their group, which includes a category of disease stabilisation (SD) as evidence of response to treatment [5]. In their definition, SD reflects no evidence of disease progression (or worsening) during the initial 12 weeks of treatment. Survival analysis of SD patients appeared to be comparable to those who had evidence of tumour regression (partial responses) during that same 12-week period and SD and PR lived significantly longer than those who did not respond (NR). These observations prompted NPCP investigators to consider SD in the category of "responding" patients together with those that demonstrated evidence of partial response. What remains unproven, however, is that stabilisation of disease was caused by treatment. Similarly, it is possible that SD patients have a relatively indolent biology and slow progression rate, which is inherent in their disease and unrelated to treatment. It is quite conceivable that those who have not demonstrated evidence of disease progression at 12 weeks will live shorter than those patients whose disease is progressing slower. Regardless of these well recognised deficiencies, the NPCP criteria for response have been widely employed and this was particularly emphasised for studies involving patients with no evidence of bidimensionally measurable disease. It should be recognised that including SD patients in the responding group may falsely inflate response rates.

The efficacy data with chemotherapy in prostate cancer is usually described by using response rates, however, because of the above factors, urological oncologists should be critical when interpreting clinical trials in

Table 2. "Alphabet Soup" of single agents studied in prostatic cancer

AMSA	ESORUBICIN	MGBG	NITROGEN MUSTARD
AZQ	ESTRACYT	ME-CCNU	PREDNIMUSTINE
BCNU	ETOPOSIDE	MELPHALAN	PROCARBAZINE
BISANTRENE	5-FU	METHOTREXATE	SPIROGERMANIUM
CCNU	GANO3	MITOMYCIN-C	STREPTOZOTOCIN
CYLOPHOSPHAMIDE	HMM	MITOXANTRONE	VINBLASTINE
CISPLATIN	HYDREA	NEOCARCINOSTATIN	VINCRISTINE
DOXORUBICIN			VINDESINE

From Eisenberger M et al. [16,25]
Abbreviations: AMSA- Amsacrine; AZQ- Azyridinylbenzoquinone; BCNU-Carmustine; CCNU-Lomustine; 5FU-5Fluorouracil; GaNO3-Gallium Nitrate; HMM-Hexamethylmelamine; MGBG-Mitoquazone

this disease. It is this author's opinion that methodological factors have a strong influence on the outcome of a study and that the variability of results observed with similar treatment programmes are largely related to the application of different methods of disease assessment.

Uncontrolled Phase II Studies

The majority of currently available drugs have been tested in patients with prostatic carcinoma (Table 2). Some of the earlier trials suffer from significant methodological problems because they represent broad phase II studies involving multiple malignancies. Such trials commonly lacked disease-oriented criteria for response and frequently included insufficient numbers of patients with the same disease. Table 3 illustrates the objective and subjective response rates and the response criteria used in the various reported series testing some of the most commonly used cytotoxic drugs.

In the analysis of these studies, it can be appreciated that there is a substantial variability in response rates reported with the same drug by different investigators. This variability cannot be adequately explained by the slight differences in dose and schedules, but most likely reflects the application of different criteria for response and/or patient selection factors. The experience with 2 widely used agents, doxorubicin and cisplatinum, clearly illustrates this problem. O'Bryan et al. [6,7] reported responses in 7/29 (29%) evaluable cases with a schedule of doxorubicin every 3 weeks in 2 broad phase II trials. However, 2 other studies using different response criteria yielded different results. Scher et al. [8], using doxorubicin every 3 weeks in patients with bidimensional measurable disease, reported only 2 complete (CR) plus partial (PR) responses (5%) in 39 evaluable cases. Torti et al. [9], using weekly low-dose doxorubicin in 25 evaluable patients, reported 4 CRs plus PRs in 12 patients with measurable disease sites, and by applying the National Prostatic Cancer Project (NPCP) criteria for response [4], observed 21 CRs plus PRs and stabilisation of disease (SD) (84%) in the 25 cases.

Merrin [10] reported 17/54 (31%) complete and partial responses and 7/54 (26%) stable disease using a weekly induction schedule of cisplatin for 6 weeks followed by maintenance every 3 weeks. These initial high response rates were not confirmed by Rossof [11], Yagoda [12] and Qazi [13] (see Table 3). While this experience, as well as those with other drugs, prevent us from drawing reliable conclusions with regard to the actual response rates for the various agents described, it is apparent that their antitumour effects are at best marginal. This information should be seriously considered prior to the selection of drugs for clinical use, especially if the treatment is associated with significant toxicity.

The same problems discussed above apply to trials reported with several multi-drug combinations evaluated (Table 4). While overall responses with some combination regimens in uncontrolled trials appear to be better than the uncontrolled data with single agents, the objective response rates (CR + PR) are still relatively low, and, furthermore, have not been shown to be superior to single agents in prospective randomised studies.

Table 3. Single-agent phase II trials in hormone-resistant prostatic carcinoma

Drug/Study	Total number of responders reported/evaluable	CR + PR	SD	Improvement[1] (subjective)	Response[2] criteria
Doxorubicin					
O'Bryan et al.	2/9	2	0	0	B
O'Bryan et al.	5/15	5	0	0	B
Torti et al.	21/25	4*	17	0	C
Blum	7/51	NR[3,4]	NR	NR	A
Scher et al.	6/39	2	1	3 (5)	D
BCNU					
Carter et al.	2/15	NR	NR	NR	A
CCNU					
Carter et al.	2/19	NR	NR	NR	A
Cyclophosphamide					
Carter et al.	8/57	NR	NR	NR	A
Cisplatin					
Yagoda et al.	4/25	3	1	0 (8)	D
Merrin	24/54	17	7	0 (20)	A
Rossof et al.	4/21	4	0	0	B
Qazi et al.	0/17	0	0	0	E
Estracyt					
Mittleman et al.	9/44	9	0	0 (7)	C
Fossa et al.	6/17	NR	NR	6 (3)	A
Jonsson et al.	28/91	NR	NR	28 (24)	A
Kuss et al.	3/15	3	0	0	A
Leistenschneider et al.	8/23	NR	NR	8 (10)	A
Edsmyr et al.	19/90[5]	NR	NR	NR (49)	A
Nilsson et al.	28/91	NR	NR	NR (24)	A
Veronesi et al.	20/27	3	17	0	C
5-Fluorouracil					
Moore et al.	7/7	4	3	0	B
Ansfield et al.	1/7	0	0	NR	B
Weiss et al.	1/4	NR	NR	NR	B
Hall et al.	3/6	NR	NR	NR (3)	B
Hydroxyurea					
Lerner et al.	19/30	15	4	0	A
Mithramycin					
Kofman et al.	2/6	NR	NR	NR	B
Carter et al.	2/36	NR	NR	NR	A
Mitomycin-C					
Humphrey et al.	0/4	0	0	0 (4)	B
Melphalan					
Houghton et al.	1/15	0	0	1 (1)	A
Nitrogen Mustard					
Karnofsky et al.	0/3	0	0	0 (2)	B
Nitrogen Mustard					
Carter et al.	12/31[4]	NR	NR	NR	A
Prednimustine					
Catane et al.	5/23	0	0	5 (8)	A
Vincristine					
Carter et al.	2/22[4]	NR	NR	NR	A

From Eisenberger M et al. [16,25]

1 Improvement - "Objective" evidence of response, but less than a PR
2 A Not specified or unclear
B Broad phase II (no specific criteria listed, or unclear)
C National Prostatic Cancer Project Response Criteria (NPCP)
D Memorial Sloan-Kettering Response Criteria
E Standard response criteria for solid tumours, including a decrease in markers
See References 5,9,16,24,25,26 for definitions of criteria for response
3 NR-Not reported (Responses reported but not quantitatively classified as CR, PR, SD or improvement)
4 Review of multiple doses/schedules
5 Included 26/90 patients with no prior hormonal treatment. Actual results for hormone-resistant patients are unclear
* 4/12 (CR + PR) in patients with bidimensionally measurable disease

Table 4. Phase II trials with combination chemotherapy

Drug/Study	Total number of responders reported/evaluable	CR + PR	SD	Improvement[1] (subjective)	Response[2] criteria
CTX + Doxorubicin					
Izbicki et al.	8/20	3	5	(8)	E
Ihde et al.	11/22	7	4		F
Merrin et al.	5/19	0	5	(8)	A
Lloyd	2/11	2	0		B
Soloway et al.	12/21	0	12	(5)	C
CTX + 5-FU					
Merrin et al.	2/13	1	1	0 (7)	A
Estramustine Phosphate + 5-FU					
Kennealy et al.	3/25	0	0	3 (8)	A
Chlorambucil + Prednisolone					
Beckley et al.	2/11	0	2	0	C
BCNU + CTX + Doxorubicin					
Presant et al.	11/27	7	4	2	E
Doxorubicin + DDP					
Citrin et al.	10/21	NR	NR	NR	G
Perloff et al.	9/17	9	0	(2)	A
CTX + Prednisolone					
Anderson et al.	7/83	NR	NR	7 (55)	A
CTX + Doxorubicin + DDP					
Seifter et al.	12/17	7	6	0	F
CTX + DDP + Prednisone					
Berry et al.	10/22	0	10	0	C
Doxorubicin + 5-FU + Mito-C					
Logothetis et al.	30/62[3]	NR	NR	NR	H
Kasimis et al.	7/16	0	7	0 (9)	C
Hsu et al.	9/14	1	8	0 (10)	C
Melphalan + MTX + 5-FU + VCR + Prednisone					
Paulson et al.	51/84[4a]	3[4b]	0	NR (40)	I
CTX + MTX + 5F-FU + VCR +Prednisone					
Buell et al.	6/16	5	1	(11)	E

From Eisenberger M. et al. [16,25]
Abbreviations: CTX- Cyclophosphamide; 5-FU - 5-Flouorouracil; DDP - Cisplatin
1 Improvement- "Objective" evidence of response, but less than a PR
2 A Not specified or unclear
B Broad phase II (no specific criteria listed, or unclear)
C National Prostatic Cancer Project Response Criteria (NPCP)
D Memorial Sloan-Kettering Response Criteria
E Standard response criteria for solid tumours, including a decrease in markers
F NCI - VAH criteria
G Citrin et al.
H Logothetis et al., M.D. Anderson Hospital and Tumour Institute
I Paulson et al.
See References, 5,9,16,24,25,26 for definitions of criteria for response
3 Responses were seen in 18/41 patients with bone metastasis only and 12/21 with bone and visceral sites (8 in the lung)
4a Twenty-four patients had at least 50 percent decrease in acid phosphatase, 13 had normalisation and 11 had ≤ 50 per cent reduction without normalisation
Twenty-seven patients had improvement in performance status correlated with improved survival
4b Three of 7 patients with bidimensionally measurable disease had CR + PR

Randomised Clinical Trials

Tables 5 and 6 show the results of most clinical trials reported during the last few years.

The NPCP tested a number of single agents and combinations in randomised trials (Table 5). By using response as the main study end-point, the NPCP initially compared single agents, cyclophosphamide and 5-Fluorouracil in NPCP Study 100, estramus-

Table 5. National Prostatic Cancer Project: Randomised trials in prostatic carcinoma

Treatment	Number evaluable/entered	CR+PR	SD	Median survival (wks)
NPCP Study 100				
CTX	41	4	20	47
5-FU	33	4	14	44
Standard	36	0	7	38
NPCP Study 200				
Estramustine Phosphate	46/54	3	11	26
Streptozotocin	38/46	0	12	25
Standard	21/25	0	4	24
NPCP Study 300				
CTX	35/39	0	9	27
DTIC	55/68	0	13	40
Procarbazine	39/58	0	5	31
NPCP Study 400				
Estramustine Phosphate+ Prednimustine	54	1	6	37 (mean)
Prednimustine	62	0	8	30 (mean)
NPCP Study 700				
CTX	43/47	3	12	41
MeCCNU	27/38	1	7	22
Hydroxyurea	28/40	2	2	19
NPCP Study 800				
Estramustine Phosphate	27/38	1	6	26
Vincristine	29/42	1	4	22
a+b	39/41	0	7	32
NPCP Study 1100				
Estramustine Phosphate	50/63	1	16	43
MTX	58/67	3	21	37
DDP	50/69	2	16	33
NPCP Study 1200				
Estramustine Phosphate	40/50	0	7	38
DDP	42/51	0	9	28
a+b	42/48	0	14	40

From Eisenberger, M. et al. [16,25]

A Radiation therapy, prednisone, TACE®, dexamethasone, testosterone, DES, stilphostrol, Aldactone®, cryosurgery, dicorvin, estinyl

tine and streptozotocin in NPCP Study 200, to a no-chemotherapy, "standard treatment", control arm [14,15,16]. The standard arm consisted of a variety of palliative treatments, such as radiation therapy, radioactive phosphorus (P 32), oestrogens, corticosteroids and analgesics only. While higher response rates were reported in the chemotherapy arms, most of these were in the stable disease category. No survival differences were seen in either study [14-16]. Despite this, the NPCP considered these 2 studies as evidence of superior benefits of chemotherapy over standard treatment for these patients and continued testing other single agents and combinations without further comparisons with a no-chemotherapy control arm. In the eight trials illustrated in Table 5, of a total of 258 "objective responders", 230 (89%) were actually included in the stable disease category. A critical evaluation of the NPCP trials would suggest that routine use of chemotherapy over "standard treatment", as defined by the group, has yet to be given stronger support.

Additional trials conducted by other groups are illustrated in Table 6. The overall results are similar to the experience reported by NPCP investigators. As indicated above, survival time in endocrine-resistant patients does not seem to be affected by the various treatments tested thus far. Table 7 illustrates the median survival times reported in phase II studies with some of the most "promising"

Table 6. Other randomised trials in prostatic carcinoma

Treatment	Number evaluable/ entered	CR + PR	SD	Improve-ment[1]	Median survival	Response[2] criteria
Smalley et al.						
5-FU	32/49	2	5	-	34 wks	A
CTX + Doxorubicin + 5-FU	39/52	2	4	-	25 wks	
Eagan et al.						
Adriamycin	19	-	-	5	NR	B
CTX + 5-FU	18	-	-	2	NR	
Chlebowski et al.						
CTX	15	0	8	-	7.2 mths	C
CTX + Doxorubicin + 5-FU	12	0	6	-	8.9 mths	
Muss et al.						
CTX	17	0	9	-	8 mths	C
CTX + MTX + 5-FU	15	1	7	-	5 mths	
Herr et al.						
CTX + MTX + 5-FU	20	3	4	-	26 wks	D
CCNU	20	0	6	-	24 wks	
Tejada et al.						
5-FU	8	2	1	-	NR	D
CCNU	10	4	2	-	NR	
Pavone-Macaluso et al.						
Doxorubicin	11/22	0	3	-	NR	C
Procarbazine	14/24	1	0	-	NR	
DeWys et al.						
Doxorubicin	96/112	15/61*	0	-	29 wks	D
5-FU	51/54	3/42*	0	-	24 wks	
Stephens et al.						
CTX + Doxorubicin	68	6/19*	18	-	27 wks	D
Hydroxyurea	69	1/24*	9	-	28 wks	
Torti et al.						
Doxorubicin	20	1/13[E]	8	-	48 wks	C
Doxorubicin + Cisplatin	17	2/10[E]	9	-	43 wks	
Kasimis et al.						
CTX	16	0	8	-	7.9 mths	C
5-FU + Doxorubicin + Mito-C	14/15	1	5	-	8.9 mths	

From Eisenberger, M. et al. [16,25]
1 Improvement reported but not quantitated, or some evidence regards as treatment benefit (decrease in marker values, decrease in prostatic size)
2 A Southeastern Cancer Study Group Criteria
B Ancillary Scoring System (including crossed-over patients)
C National Prostatic Cancer Project Criteria
D Usual criteria for solid tumours, including a decrease in acid phosphatase
E Objective responses in patients with measurable disease. Because of this the denominators of total entered and evaluable is different
See References 5,9,16,24,25,26 for definitions of response criteria
* Patients with "measurable disease" only (including bidimensionally measurable disease, elevated markers or presence of "evaluable" bony lesions). Figures include crossed-over patients
NR-Not Reported

regimens, producing response rates (CR + PR + SD) of 20% or better. These survival figures are well within the range observed in all other studies and, moreover, are comparable to the 2 no-chemotherapy (standard treatment) control arms of NPCP studies 100 and 200. The Kaplan-Meyer survival curves of all NPCP studies in Table 5 and the studies described in Table 6 are shown in Figures 1 and 2. Figure 3 depicts all survival curves of contemporary randomised studies with 20 or more patients per arm. The importance of Figure 3 is that not only does it demonstrate that survival of endocrine-resistant patients entered into prospective trials is short, but also that the curve distributions of social studies follow a relatively narrow range, suggesting that survival has not been affected in any major way by any of the treatments tested. It is also important to recognise that,

Table 7. Survival figures available in phase II trials with ≥ 20 percent CR + PR + SD

Drug	Response rate	Median survival (weeks)		
		All evaluable patients	Responders	
Doxorubicin	84% (21/25)	41	--	
Estramustine phosphate	20% (9/44)	--	40	
Estramustine phosphate	35% (6/17)	16	--	
CTX + Doxorubicin	50% (11/22)	44	56 44	(CR+PR - 7pts) (SD - 4 pts)
CTX + Doxorubicin	40% (8/20)	--	40	
CTX + Doxorubicin + 5-FU	57% (12/21)	--	40	
BCNU + CTX + Doxorubicin	40% (11/27)	--	36	
CTX + DDP + Prednisone	45% (10/22)	36	40	
Doxorubicin + 5-FU + Mito C	48% (30/62)	--	47.5	
Doxorubicin + 5-FU + Mito C	44% (7/16)	--	48	
Doxorubicin + 5-FU + Mito C	64% (9/14)	--	33	

From Eisenberger M. et al. [16]

among the curves included in this graph, are the "standard treatment" control arms of NPCP studies 100 and 200.

Combined Chemo-Endocrine Treatment as the Initial Systemic Approach

More recently, much attention has been focussed on defining the optimal timing for treatment with cytotoxic drugs in cancer of the prostate. Data derived from preclinical experiments in the Dunning adenocarcinoma tumour model indicates that this tumour is comprised of hormonally dependent and independent cell clones (tumour cell heterogeneity) [17]. Experiments using androgen ablation and/or chemotherapy in this tumour model suggest that early combined therapy may be superior to treatment with either modality alone, or applied in any other sequence. Unfortunately, however, while antitumour mechanisms and effects with endocrine treatment in the Dunning tumour model are somewhat comparable with human prostate cancer, the same is not true with non-hormonal chemotherapeutic agents. Cautious extrapolation of data with chemotherapy between species should be undertaken primarily because the results with this modality in the Dunning tumour model have not been reproducible in prostate cancer in man. Nonetheless, since tumour progression following gonadal ablation reflects to a great extent an expansion of previously existing endocrine-independent clones, the use of combined endocrine and non-endocrine treatment as the initial approach has a sound theoretical rationale, and early initiation of combined treatment may be more effective when the tumour burden is smaller.
This, however, has not been confirmed by existing clinical data. Clinical trials combining

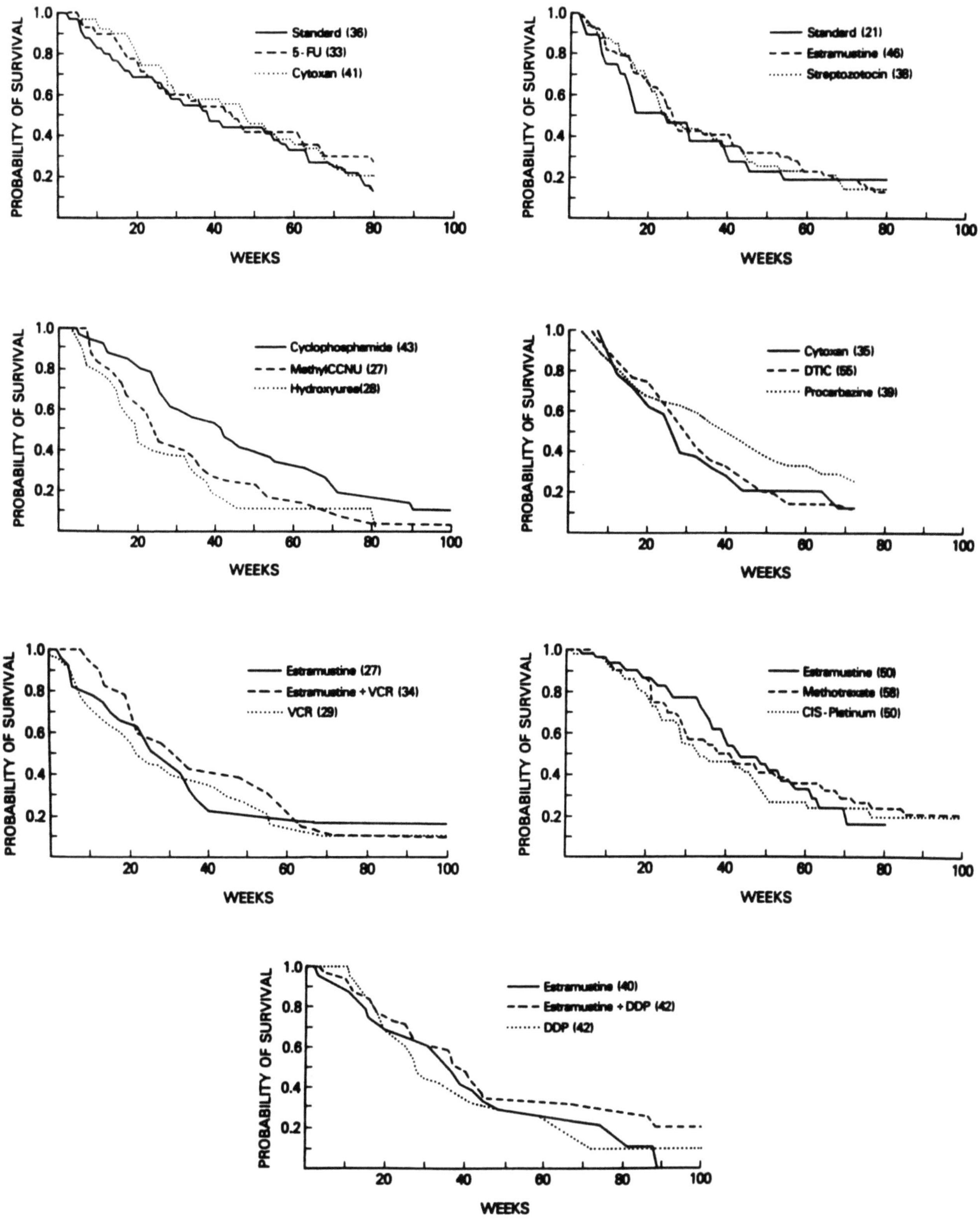

Fig. 1. Survival of NPCP chemotherapy studies

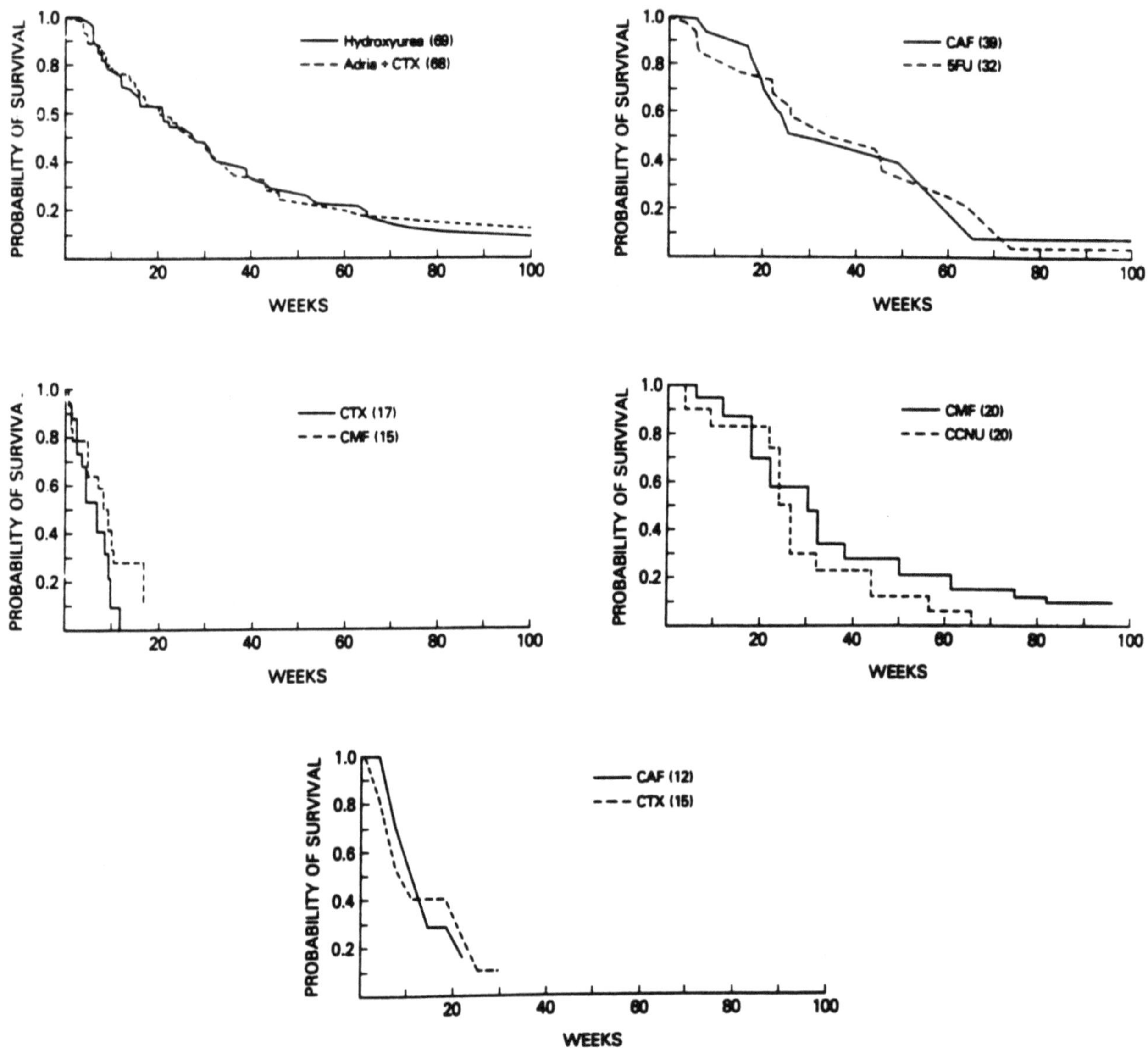

Fig. 2. Survival of other chemotherapy trials (non-NPCP)

chemotherapy plus endocrine treatment have focused primarily on patients with stage D_2 disease without prior systemic treatment.

The National Prostatic Cancer Project conducted two randomised trials, one in newly diagnosed stage D_2 patients comparing diethylstilboestrol (DES) or orchiectomy versus DES plus cyclophosphamide versus cyclophosphamide plus estramustine phosphate (NPCP #500) and another comparing DES, DES plus cyclophosphamide or DES plus estramustine phosphate in stable patients on initial hormonal therapy (NPCP #600) [18,19].

The Southeastern Cancer Study Group conducted a trial comparing DES alone to DES plus cyclophosphamide in newly diagnosed stage D_2 patients. Preliminary results of this study did not demonstrate any advantage for the combination arm [20]. A follow-up report has not been published at this time.

The Southwest Oncology Group has conducted a study comparing orchiectomy alone to orchiectomy plus the combination of cyclophosphamide and doxorubicin, however, the results of this trial still have to be published.

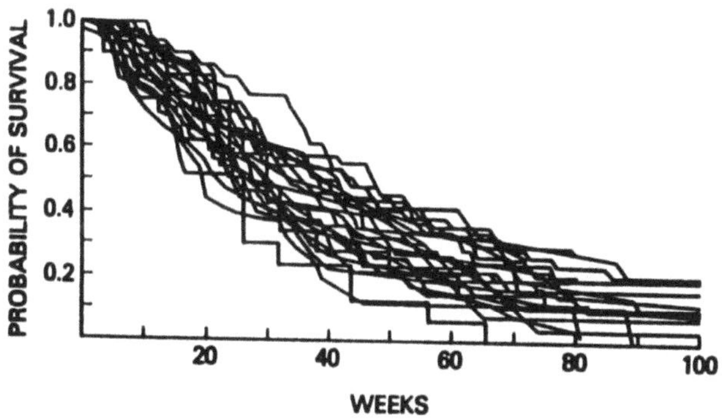

Fig. 3. Composite graph of survival curves of all studies with 20 or more patients per arm

The median survival curves of all randomised studies with combined endocrine/chemotherapy are comparable to those reported in the VA studies (VACURG) more than 2 decades ago and also to more recent studies with various endocrine treatments alone in patients with stage D_2 disease [1,2].
The administration of exogenous testosterone for priming prostate cancer cells and therefore increasing their susceptibility to chemotherapy has also been explored [21,22]. Manni et al. [22] studied this approach in 85 patients with endocrine-resistant disease, all of whom had an orchiectomy followed by adrenal androgen suppression with aminoglutethimide and hydrocortisone. All patients were randomised to receive exogenous androgen treatment with combination chemotherapy or combination chemotherapy alone, and the results showed no advantage in response rates, time to progression or survival. These negative results may be at least partly explained by the selection of patients with endocrine-resistant (or androgen-independent) disease who may have been only minimally susceptible to exogenous androgenic stimulation, even though some increase in toxicity was reported in the stimulation arm. Similarly, the lack of significant antitumour activity observed with chemotherapy in both arms suggests that this study did not constitute optimal conditions for testing this interesting approach.
More recently, Huben et al. [23] reported on a trial with stage 2 patients randomly allocated to receive treatment with DES or orchiectomy, Buserelin (LHRH analogue) or DES or orchiectomy plus methotrexate (MTX). The authors report a significant difference in time to progression in favour of DES/orchiectomy with and without MTX over the LHRH arm, but no differences in survival, even though median survival figures had not been reached for all arms. They conclude that the shorter time to progression on Buserelin may be explained by the initial "flare" phenomenon observed with LHRH analogue treatment. This phenomenon could result in a higher incidence of early progressions and therefore shorten the overall median time to progression for the entire group.
In summary, the results of these studies have not supported the usefulness of combined chemo-endocrine approaches, however, it may be argued that this is not completely surprising in view of the lack of efficacy of the chemotherapeutic agents available thus far. While routine use of combined treatment with conventional cytotoxic drugs and endocrine manipulations cannot be justified at this time, this approach remains a viable option for future research with new systemic treatments for this disease.

Current Recommendations and Future Considerations

The management of endocrine-resistant patients represents a major dilemma to practising urological oncologists. The important issue to be recognised is that current means of treatment have not been shown to prolong survival, thus the main objective is to palliate symptoms and maintain reasonable levels of quality of life.
Based on the data described here, some management recommendations can be made. Continuous support to research institutions committed to developing new forms of treatment should receive highest priority; as such, it also provides patients with the opportunity to receive new forms of treatment which ultimately may prove to be effective. Outside of the research environment, the administration of second-line endocrine approaches, in addition to the usual palliative procedures (radiation therapy to painful areas and analgesia), is a reasonable approach, especially in view of their acceptable tolerance and

therefore favourable therapeutic index. Corticosteroids have been widely employed and have been shown to result in subjective benefits in a proportion of patients. When all above measures have failed to provide appropriate palliation, the use of conventional cytotoxic chemotherapy may be considered. There is no justification in employing multidrug combinations as opposed to single agents. Among the single agents we recommend cyclophosphamide, methotrexate, doxorubicin, or 5-fluorouracil. If such treatment is undertaken, the drug of choice should be selected judiciously with specific attention to its toxicity pattern.

Much has been written with regard to the disease process itself, but the status of the host is also of major importance. The overwhelming majority of the patients included in the chemotherapy trials described in this review had far advanced disease and were extensively pretreated. Such characteristics, coupled with the usual limitations in performance status, are strong adverse factors with regard to chances for effective palliation. Despite these well recognised limitations, urological oncologists still reserve chemotherapy for those patients who have become refractory to first-line and many times second- and third-line endocrine treatments and usually are given palliative radiation to various painful areas. The experience derived from other, more chemosensitive, tumours strongly supports the view that extent of prior treatment, performance status and extent of disease are among the strongest prognostic indicators for outcome in therapeutic trials. Thus, the poor results observed with chemotherapy thus far may, at least partly, be explained by the selection of a group of patients with adverse features, who are unlikely to respond to any treatment.

The palliative and long-term results with endocrine treatment in patients with far advanced stage D_2 are significantly worse than those observed in patients with lesser tumour burden. This probably reflects the presence of an already substantial proportion of androgen-independent tumour clones in those patients with extensive tumour burden. While the poor response to cytotoxic treatment is in great part a function of its relative inefficacy against this disease, some theoretical considerations can be entertained such as: 1) the mechanisms involved in the development of endocrine resistance may have an important role in resistance to cytotoxic treatment; 2) as with endocrine treatment, response to cytotoxic chemotherapy may be less likely in more advanced and heavily pretreated patients; 3) as in other more responsive tumour types (such as testis cancer, lymphomas, breast cancer, small-cell lung cancer), the magnitude of response to treatment may be proportional to the initial tumour burden. Such hypothetical considerations may be evaluated clinically by treating selected, newly diagnosed stage D_2 patients with chemotherapy prior to endocrine treatment (such as those with poor prognostic features and measurable disease). This should obviously be done in a strictly controlled and investigational setting. In a preliminary trial reported by Seifter et al. [24], 17 patients with newly diagnosed stage D_2 disease received a combination of cyclophosphamide, doxorubicin and cisplatin before endocrine treatment was given. This approach was shown to be feasible and to produce some responses. In our opinion, such investigational therapeutic intervention is ethically and scientifically justified since it has not been shown conclusively that early androgen ablation results in survival advantages over delayed treatment at the time patients become symptomatic. This is particularly the case with those asymptomatic patients with extensive stage D_2 disease in whom survival is usually short and significantly worse than in those with relatively limited metastatic disease. This concept offers a new avenue for testing promising new agents under potentially better conditions.

REFERENCES

1 Byar DP: The Veterans Administration Cooperative Urological Research Group's studies of cancer of the prostate. Cancer 1973 (32):1126-1130
2 The Leuprolide Study Group: Leuprolide versus diethylstilbestrol for metastatic prostatic cancer. N Engl J Med 1984 (311):1281-1286
3 Isaacs JT, Isaacs WB et al: Establishment and characterization of seven Dunning rat prostatic cancer cell lines and their use in developing methods for predicting metastatic abilities of prostatic cancer. The Prostate 1986 (9):261-281
4 Isaacs JT, Coffey DS: Adaptation versus selection on the mechanism responsible for the relapse of prostatic cancer to androgen ablation therapy studied in the Dunning R-3327-H adenocarcinoma. Cancer Res 1981 (41):5070-5075
5 Slack NH, Mittleman A, Brady MF, Murphy GP, and investigators in the National Prostatic Cancer Project: The importance of the stable category for chemotherapy treated patients with advanced and relapsing prostate cancer. Cancer 1980 (46):2393-2402
6 O'Bryan RM, Luce JK, Talley RW, Gottlieb JF, Baker L, Bonadonna G: Phase II evaluation of adriamycin in human neoplasia. Cancer 1973 (32):1-8
7 O'Bryan RM, Baker LH, Gottlieb JF, Rivkin SE, Balcerzak SP, Grumet GN, Salmon SE, Moon TE, Hoogstraten B: Dose-response evaluation of adriamycin in human neoplasia. Cancer 1977 (39):1940-1948
8 Scher H, Yagoda A, Watson R, Serber M, Whitmore W: Phase II trial of adriamycin in bidimensionally measurable prostatic adenocarcinoma. J Urol 1984 (13):1099-1102
9 Torti F, Aston D, Lum BL, Kohler M, Williams R, Spaulding JT, Shortliffe LD, Freiha FS: Weekly doxorubicin in endocrine refractory carcinoma of the prostate. J Clin Oncol 1983 (1/8):477-482
10 Merrin C: Treatment of genitourinary tumors with cis-dichloro diamine platinum (II). Experience in 250 patients. Cancer Treat Rep 1979 (63):1578-1589
11 Rossof AH, Talley RW, Stephens R, Thigpen T, Samson M, Groppe C, Eyre HJ, Eisher R: Phase II evaluation of cis-dichloro diamine platinum (II) in advanced malignancies of the genitourinary and gynecological organs: A Southwest Oncology Group Study. Cancer Treat Rep 1979 (63):1557-1564
12 Yagoda A, Watson RC, Natale RB, Barzell W, Sogani P, Grabstald H, Whitmore W: A critical analysis of response criteria in patients with prostatic cancer treated with cisdiaminedichloro platinum II. Cancer 1979 (4):1553-1562
13 Qazi R, Khandekar J: Phase II study of cisplatin for metastatic prostatic carcinoma. An Eastern Cooperative Oncology Group Study. Am J Clin Oncol (CCT) 1983 (6):203-205
14 Scott WW, Gibbons RP, Johnson DE, Prout GR, Schmidt JD, Saroff J, Murphy GP: The continued evaluation of the effects of chemotherapy in patients with advanced carcinoma of the prostate. J Urol 1976 (116):211-213
15 Murphy GP, Gibbons RP, Johnson DE, Loening SA, Prout GR, Schmidt JD, Bross DS, Chu TM, Gaeta J, Saroff J: A comparison of estramustine phosphate and streptozotocin in patients with prostatic carcinoma who had extensive irradiation. J Urol 1977 (118):288-291
16 Eisenberger M, Simon R, O'Dwyer P, Wittes R, Friedman M: A re-evaluation of non-hormonal cytotoxic chemotherapy in treatment of prostatic carcinoma. J Clin Oncol 1985 (3):827-841
17 Isaacs JT: The timing of androgen ablation therapy and/or chemotherapy in the treatment of prostatic cancer.
18 Murphy GP, Beckley S, Brady MF, Chu M, Dekernion J, Dhabuwala C, Gaeta JF, Gibbons RP and NRCP investigators: Treatment of newly diagnosed prostate cancer patients with chemotherapy agents in combination with hormones versus hormones alone. Cancer 1983 (51):1264-1277
19 Gibbons RP, Beckley S, Brady MF, Chu TM, Dekernion JB, Dhabuwala C, Gaeta FJ, Leoning SA, McKiel CR, McLeod DG, Pontes JE, Prout GR, Scardino PT, Schlegel IV, Schmidt JU, Scott WW, Slack NJ, Soloway MS, Murphy GP: The addition of chemotherapy to hormonal therapy for treatment of patients with metastatic carcinoma of the prostate. J Surg Oncol 1983 (23):133-142
20 Moore M: Chemohormonal therapy for stage D prostatic cancer. Preliminary results of a randomized trial. Am Soc Clin Oncol 1982 abstr C-461
21 Kedia KR, Kellermeyer RW: Hormonal stimulation followed by multiagent chemotherapy in advanced prostatic cancer. Cancer Chemoth Pharmacol 1982 (18):261-265
22 Manni A, Bartholomew M, Caplan R, Boucher A, Santen R, Lipron A, Harvey H, Simmonds M, White-Hershey D, Gordon R: Androgen priming and chemotherapy in advanced prostate cancer: evaluation of determinants of clinical outcome. J Clin Oncol 1988 (6):1456-1466
23 Huben RP, Murphy GP and NPCP investigators: A comparison of DES/orchiectomy with Buserelin and with methotrexate plus DES and orchiectomy in newly diagnosed patients with clinical stage D2 cancer of the prostate. Cancer 1988 (62):1881-1887
24 Seifter E, Bunn P, Cohen M, Ihde D: A trial of combination chemotherapy followed by therapy for previously untreated metastatic carcinoma of the prostate. J Clin Oncol 1984 (4):1305-1373
25 Eisenberger MA, Abrams JS: Chemotherapy for prostatic carcinoma. Sem Urol 1988 (6):303-310
26 Yagoda A: Response in prostate cancer: An enigma. Sem Urol 1984 (1):311-319

Current Trends of Treatment

Louis Denis

Department of Urology, Algemeen Ziekenhuis Middelheim, Lindendreef 1, 2020 Antwerp, Belgium

Cancer of the prostate represents 10% of all cancers in males and recently became the second most frequent cancer in men in the industrial nations of West Europe and North America. This increase in incidence and mortality is small but real. The greying of the male population and the increasing detection of localised cancer by new technology probably account for most of this increase. The most recent survey of prostate cancer, organised by the American College of Surgeons, showed that close to 50% of the newly diagnosed cases presented with localised disease [1]. This exceptional change in trend to earlier diagnosis is due to increased awareness on the part of urologists and patients alike in the search for locally confined cancer. Also high-risk patients selected by transrectal ultrasound and/or elevated prostate cancer markers are more frequently diagnosed by ultrasound-guided biopsy. This fortuitous situation is somewhat offset by the lack of consensus on preferred treatment, as revealed in a symposium organised by the National Institutes of Health of the USA [2].

This lack of treatment consensus is also present in the more advanced stages of disease, although endocrine treatment is the established first-line treatment. The ESO Task Force on the medical management of prostatic cancer confirmed in 1988 an uneven distribution of patterns of care in Europe [3]. This uncertainty in treatment choice may reflect the heterogeneous presentation of prostatic cancer in the older males ranging from a microscopic form of cancer to a symptomatic metastatic cancer. There is agreement that the earliest form of the disease is the prostate intra-epithelial neoplasia (PIN). These lesions are not only associated with prostate cancer but are thought to develop into cancer. Here a distinction has to be made between focal and diffuse forms of cancer. Both of these forms are called latent (awaiting development into a clinical form) or incidental (discovered by the pathologist in surgical or autopsy specimens), but they have a very different prognosis. The small focal lesions, with well-differentiated histology, invading a minimal amount of tissue, grow slowly and progress to invasion in only 2% of the cases over a 4-year period [4]. The diffuse lesions, with a greater tumour volume and, usually, poorly differentiated histology, progress to invasion in 30% of the cases during the same period. Both forms develop into the clinical form of cancer where detection is possible by palpation or imaging technology, of which transrectal ultrasound is the most popular at this moment. Symptomatology quite naturally is caused by the local or metastatic tumour mass. Again, differentiation of the cell and tumour volume determine the outcome of the disease. The concept that increased tumour mass defines differentiation and prognosis also prevails in node-positive disease as well as in the final stages of bone metastatic disease. This universal concept of continuous tumour growth is clearly recognised in the nodal stages of the TNM classification [5]. Node-negative patients do far better than node-positive patients in the time to invasive disease ($p < 0.00005$) [6] and patients with lesser metastatic tumour burden live longer than patients with extensive disease [7]. Prostate cancer is one single biological entity with a constant growth rate, where a strong correlation exists between tumour volume and cell differentiation [8]. It is thus quite logical that these 2 factors are the 2 most powerful prognostic factors that bear on progression of disease and survival.

Aspects of Treatment Decisions

Natural History

Effective treatment should, by definition, improve the natural course of the disease and the effects should increase the time to progression, increase survival and provide a better overall quality of life for the patient. It is extremely difficult to prove these points in randomised clinical trials for several reasons. The first reason is, of course, that most forms of clinical cancer are treated, which leaves us with the treated natural history. The second reason is that prostate cancer covers a wide spectrum of disease and one should make a distinction between incidental, localised, node positive, minimal metastatic and extensive metastatic disease. A final category is endocrine-treated prostate cancer, which is wholly, or partly, refractory to the given endocrine treatment. This form of disease is usually called prostate cancer in relapse. The third reason is, that some prognostic factors, such as histological differentiation, have more effect on the course of disease than the usual endocrine treatment. The fourth reason is that many other causes of death influence the outcome of the disease. The fifth, but not the least important reason, is that most randomised trials by limiting themselves to a few hundred patients can only detect statistical differences to the range of a 20% improvement in median time to survival which can hardly be expected in almost identical treatments. An additional problem is the fact that data collection and analysis requires a concerted effort from a large number of people subject to rigorous quality control.

The most striking event in the natural history of prostate cancer is the enormous difference in incidence between the focal cancers, found in autopsy material, as compared to the local clinical tumour still confined to the prostate. Depending on the age group, only one clinical cancer is found for every 80 to 500 incidental cancers. In general, one may state that the malignant potential increases with time, and a strong correlation is present between actual tumour volume and capsule penetration, seminal vesicle invasion and metastatic disease [8]. The time to progression or invasion depends largely on the cell differentiation where moderately or poorly differentiated cancers show an increase in aggressive tumour activity. This explains the abundance of advanced, disseminated disease as compared to the locally confined cancerous nodule and their very different survival rates.

Treatment aimed at the locally confined disease by radical prostatectomy or transurethral resection and endocrine therapy in 1963 [9], or placebo [10], established that there were no remarkable differences in survival over 10 and 15 years of follow-up for this type of tumour. No wonder that it was equally difficult 2 decades later to show survival differences in patients with local disease treated by radical surgery or external beam irradiation [2]. In contrast, median survival in treated patients with locally invasive, node-positive disease decreases to a median of 7 years [11], where the median survival in patients with metastatic disease hovers around 2.5 years in clinical trials [12]. The worst final stage of the disease, prostate cancer in relapse, leaves the patient a median 6-month survival with a poor quality of life [13].

Our limited knowledge of the natural history of the disease calls for restraint in aggressive therapy in the older patients and leaves us waiting for the results of randomised trials with a control - no treatment - arm and early versus delayed endocrine treatment [14].

Histological Grade

The histological diagnosis and grading rests essentially on the degree of cellular anaplasia and the glandular structure of the provided tissue specimen. Over 40 grading systems have been advocated, but the Gleason grading system is widely accepted [15]. However, wide variations in grading between different pathologists are evident and the usual specimen, a core prostatic biopsy, is rarely representative of the total tumour histology. Aspiration biopsy focussing on the cellular variability, or DNA ploidy studies, may overcome this very real problem. There is, however, consensus that once poorly differentiated tumours are diagnosed, a worse prognosis is to be expected. Central pathology is a must in clinical research and automated studies with telepathological consultation will be the routine in the future.

Diagnosis

The diagnosis of prostate cancer in daily praxis is based on the suspected induration and/or asymmetry of the gland detected by rectal examination. Subsequent biopsy will be positive in half of these cases. On other occasions, one is confronted with a patient with elevated prostate cancer markers in the serum, osteoblastic bone lesions on imaging examinations, or suggestive histology in biopsy specimens taken from unidentified tumours elsewhere in the body.
The simplicity of the rectal examination is deceptive since graphic reproductions of palpation vary considerably with time whether carried out by the same examiner or, more certainly, by different examiners [16].
Ultrasound technology has completely changed the urological clinic: transrectal ultrasound, in particular, produces reliable and reproducible documentation on the volume of the prostate, its general shape and symmetry, its delineation against the surrounding tissues, as well as a detailed view of its internal echoes at different levels of the gland. Ultrasound is by far the most reliable imaging technique in comparison with other imaging techniques, including computed tomography (CT) and nuclear magnetic resonance (NMR) [17]. The consensus is that by using the more advanced technology in experienced hands, clinical prostate cancer can be defined and staged, while ultrasound-guided biopsy is superior to digitally guided biopsy. However, the value of transrectal ultrasonography as an independent screening procedure in asymptomatic patients has not yet been established. In conclusion, one may state that digital rectal examination in combination with ultrasound guided transrectal biopsy is an excellent basis for the diagnosis of cancer, staging it properly and estimating the prostate cancer volume in the majority of cases [18].

Staging

Once having established the diagnosis, one has to verify the true extent of the disease. There are no tests sensitive or specific enough to be used as a screening marker, but prostate specific antigen (PSA) has established its superiority over prostatic acid phosphatase in monitoring response and ability to predict prognosis in patients with prostate cancer [19].
However, highly increased values of PSA over 40 g/ml are indicative of metastatic disease. The first examinations include bone scan, ultrasonography of the liver, a chest X-ray and an intravenous pyelography. Close to half of the patients have metastatic disease, which eliminates the need for nodal evaluation by computed tomography. Surgical pelvic lymphadenectomy is only indicated when radical surgery and/or external beam radiation in certain instances is contemplated. The tumour can be classified in the TNM system which has been adopted as the universal staging system after the metastatic and nodal classifications are established. The system tries to follow similar approaches to all solid tumour systems to obtain a simple classification, based on minimal, localised, advanced and metastatic disease serving clinical and pathological classifications alike. This new system has met with criticism in the subdivision of extraprostatic tumour classification and clinical studies are organised to provide data to support or refute this aspect of classification [20]. The clinical staging procedures are presented in Table 1.
The presence or absence of metastatic disease is the most important prognostic factor. As cited, the prevalent osteoblastic bone metastases are best detected by bone scan. The rare soft tissue metastases to liver, lung or retroperitoneum are best detected by computed tomography. Highly elevated serum markers for prostate cancer with a negative bone scan require a more extended search for metastases. Moderate elevations of serum markers may be due to local or nodal disease, concurrent benign prostatic hyperplasia, or to rectal examinations or prostatic infarct. Under- and overstaging of local extracapsular disease will be limited by adequate use of guided biopsies. Next, the TNM grade and stage, high serum levels of PSA, low serum testosterone levels and poor performance status with anaemia due to cancer, have all been recognised as factors

Table 1. Scheme of routine staging procedures

Digital rectal examination:	DRE
Biopsy procedures:	Core needle Fine needle (quadrant) Transurethral prostatectomy* Node aspiration*
Imaging:	Intravenous pyelography Transrectal ultrasound Computed tomography*/ Nuclear magnetic resonance*
Urological procedures:	Cystoscopy Lymphadenectomy
Markers:	Prostate-specific antigen Prostatic acid phosphatase Alkaline phosphatase

* optional

that closely correlate to prognosis in the individual patient.

Clinical Research

The prime objective of our clinical research is the quest for new drugs active against hormone-independent prostate cancer cells. The ongoing phase I/II studies concentrate on safety, toxicity and therapeutical efficacy in measurable disease. Measurable disease as utilised by the urological group of the European Organisation on Research and Treatment of Cancer (EORTC) and response criteria to measure effective treatment as measurable or evaluable are presented in Table 2.

It is appropriate to remember that the primary tumour may react quite differently from metastatic tumours with regard to response rate and duration of response [21]. The consensus proposal, discussed in the 1989 meeting organised by the EORTC GU Group to assess the primary tumour, included the recommendation to adopt the 1987 TNM system; a categorisation with the inclusion of representative grading as appropriate, biopsy preferred to transurethral resection, digital rectal examinations should be recorded, transrectal ultrasound is able to differentiate T2 from T3 lesions, and CT/NMR do not contribute essentially to the T-stage. The TNM category and grade are presented in Table 3. The criteria for objective, evaluable responses are not clearly established and vary among the different clinical groups. Efforts to reach consensus on these variables resulted in various meetings organised by the American Cancer Society (USA) and the EORTC, where randomised studies on prostate cancer were analysed [22]. They established the value of prognostic factors and provided proof that these factors were more decisive in the outcome of the disease than endocrine therapy. Some of these factors are presented in Table 4. The conclusion is that stratification for patient and disease characteristics is essential to a meaningful analysis. Thus, randomised trials require large numbers of patients with adequate quality control on data collection and statistical methodology to allow comparisons be-

Table 2. Response cirteria in prostatic cancer

Measurable	Evaluable	
Nodal masses	Primary tumour Hot spots on bone scan	Performance status Pain
Nodular lung metastases	Ureteral dilatation	Weight
Nodular liver metastases	Bone metastases on X-ray Haemoglobin PSA (prostate specific antigen) Liver function tests	Urological symptoms
Objective	Objective	Subjective

Table 3. Summary prostate cancer TNM categorisation

Classification	
T1	Incidental finding
T1a	≤ 3 foci
T1b	> 3 foci
T2	Present clinically or grossly, limited to gland
T2a	≤1.5 cm
T2b	>1.5 cm/ > one lobe
T3	Invades prostatic apex/beyond capsule/ bladder neck/ seminal vesicle/not fixed
T4	Fixed or invades other adjacent structures
N1	Single ≤ 2 cm
N2	Single > 2 cm ≤ 5 cm, multiple ≤ 5 cm
N3	> 5 cm
Grade	
GX	Grade cannot be assessed
G1	Well differentiated, slight anaplasia
G2	Moderately differentiated, moderate anaplasia
G3-4	Poorly differentiated or undifferentiated marked anaplasia

tween results of randomised trials. Since very few trials, if any, fulfill these strict criteria, a major effort between all trial groups has been launched to examine the possibility of a meta-analysis of prostate cancer randomised trials involving combination treatment [23]. This policy will give us a chance to detect treatment effects which may be smaller than the usual 20% differences.

Choice of Treatment

It is generally accepted that 60-80% of the patients derive some benefit from first-line endocrine treatment. However, complete responses are rare, and even patients with partial objective responses progress after a median time of 18 to 24 months to a refractory state to endocrine treatment.

Table 4. Prognostic factors for duration of survival (all causes of death) in decreasing order of prognostic significance in patients with M1 disease: variables retained in Cox's ph model using a step-down procedure (EORTC 30761-30762)

Highly significant ($p < 0.001$)	Performance states Alkaline phosphatase Serum testosterone
Significant ($p < 0.05$)	Acid phosphatase
Marginally ($p < 0.01$)	Haemoglobin Treatment

It is also accepted that patients with N2-3 and M1 disease are not suitable for locoregional treatment and most urologists believe that T4, with reservations for T3, and N1-3 positive disease have systemic disease and are beyond cure.

The most important immediate goal is to stimulate the trend to earlier diagnosis where cure is still possible in most patients. A few screening studies are in progress to evaluate transrectal ultrasonography and/or prostate specific antigen in the early diagnosis of prostate cancer. There is no other systemic treatment available which comes close to the objective and subjective responses obtained by endocrine therapy or, for that matter, which shows reliable therapeutical effect in more than a marginal number of patients. The only exception remains estramustine phosphate which is in reality a combination treatment with endocrine and chemotherapeutic components. The search for new drugs active against prostate cancer is the next most important goal of our clinical research. This type of treatment is indicated in patients with endocrine refractory disease and in patients with poor prognostic factors at initial diagnosis. The third goal is to provide endocrine treatment which is palliative in nature to improve the quality of life of the patient for the duration of the response.

There are only 3 questions to consider in the choice of first-line endocrine treatment: the timing of the treatment, which endocrine treatment and alternative/additional treatment.

Early or Differed Endocrine Treatment

There is no clear answer to this question at the moment and one must realise that "early" in this context really means late treatment. Two randomised EORTC studies are open in which patients with proven node-positive disease or patients without symptoms and prostate cancer T1-T3 N_X M_0 at initial diagnosis are randomised to immediate hormonal treatment, or differed treatment at the time of progressive disease. Progressive disease includes, quite naturally, objective and subjective progression.

Another study, initiated by the urological group of the Medical Research Council, randomises patients with advanced asymptomatic disease between immediate and differed bilateral orchiectomy [24].

These concepts are different from the studies which try to evaluate the role of endocrine therapy in localised disease as neo-adjuvant or adjuvant therapy.

Choice of First-Line Hormonal Treatment

The 2 main principles of endocrine treatment at this moment attempt to suppress androgen production or to block the effect of circulating androgens at the level of the prostate cancer cell. The various current first-line treatments are presented in Table 5.

Bilateral orchiectomy is still the accepted standard by most urologists. This simple surgery removes in effect 95% of the total testosterone production by elimination of the Leydig cells. The morbidity is acceptable from a general point of view but the majority of patients, if given a choice, prefer medical castration. The stigma of castration can, however, be avoided by the subcapsular technique where only the functional part of the testicle is removed.

Medical castration is obtained by interference with the pituitary gonadal axis, by decreasing the luteotrophic hormone by means of oestrogenic hormones or luteotropic hormone re-

Table 5. First-line endocrine treatment

Androgen deprivation	
Surgical castration	Bilateral orchiectomy Subcapsular bilateral orchiectomy
Medical castration	Oestrogens diethylstilboestrol 1 mg polyoestradiolphosphate 160 mg i.m. LHRH agonists depot preparations goserelin 3.6 ng s.c.
Androgen blockade	
Steroid anti-androgens	Cyproterone-acetate
Pure anti-androgens	Flutamide 3 x 250 mg/day Nilutamide 2 x 150 mg/day Casodex 50 mg/day
Combination treatment	
Maximal androgen withdrawal	LHRH A depot and anti-androgens Bilateral orchiectomy and anti-androgens
Combinations endocrine/chemotherapy	Estramustine phosphate 560-840 mg/day

leasing hormone agonists (LHRHA). The oestrogens also raise the sex-hormone binding globulin (SHBG) and may exert an antitumoural effect at the prostate cellular level [25]. Diethylstilboestrol (DES) has been extensively used in doses ranging from 5 to 1 mg per day. Although several studies have confirmed its efficacy with regard to orchiectomy and its superiority in lowering cancer death over placebo, the significant cardiovascular toxicity and associated mortality eliminated the 3 and 5 mg daily dose from consideration for routine treatment [26]. The DES 1 mg per day was proven to be effective in an EORTC randomised trial against bilateral orchiectomy. This dose, with monitoring of serum testosterone (T) for efficacy and the cardiovascular status for toxicity, offers an alternative choice. A lower dose does not only diminish cardiovascular toxicity, but also parenteral forms of oestrogens, as shown in a randomised trial of Finnprostata, were quite free of these side effects. As a matter of fact, changes introduced in the serum lipoprotein lipids by parenteral polyoestradiol phosphate (160 mg per month) seemed to decrease the role of atherosclerosis [27]. These observations should be followed in larger numbers of patients. A combination compound, estramustine phosphate, an association of oestradiol with nitrogen mustard, exerts an antigonadotrophin and a cytotoxic effect. The latter effect is explained by the specific binding to the microtubular-associated proteins in the cancer cells. Its use is advocated in poorly differentiated cancer [28]. The ability of the LHRH analogues, when given in adequate doses over a period of time, to desensitise the pituitary LH-producing cells by downregulation, results in medical castration by lowering the LH secretion. No side effects were noted in the many phase II and phase III studies reported with the LHRH A treatment in its many presentations as daily injections, pernasal absorption, or monthly depot injections [29]. There is a general trend towards the depot preparations for reasons of bio-availability and for practical reasons [30]. All LHRH A share the property of stimulating LH secretion following initial administration.

This results in the rise of serum T for the next 3 days. This transient rise of serum T may provoke increased bone pain, a rise in the tumour markers and complication of spinal cord compression or ureteral obstruction in patients with extensive disease. A short concomitant therapy of oestrogens, anti-androgens or ketoconazole will block these complications. Otherwise, the LHRH A lack any toxicity, except the physiological results of T deprivation. An interesting aspect of this treatment is its complete reversibility after stopping the treatment. This property obliges the disciplined administration of the drug to avoid intermittent exacerbations of serum T, but it also allows a trial period to check whether the specific cancer is hormone sensitive [31]. Identical response rates as compared to oestrogens or bilateral orchiectomy have been reported [32]. Several studies on the patient's preference towards surgical or medical castration showed a definite trend in favour of medical castration.

According to published data, one may assume that bilateral orchiectomy is an adequate therapy as compared to depot LHRH A implantations and surgical as well as medical castration is acceptable as state-of-the-art therapy. The fact that oestrogen therapy in elevated doses has been shown in some studies to increase the time to progression, although offset by its cardiovascular toxicity, revives the hypothesis of a direct cytotoxic effect [33,34]. Progesterone compounds have been utilised, especially medroxyprogesterone acetate (MPA) and chlormadinone acetate (MDA), however, with cardiovascular toxicity present and a decreased rate in response and survival.

The anti-androgens, in contrast to all these regimens, only block the androgen receptors in the presence of normal or elevated levels of testosterone. There are 2 types of anti-androgens: the steroidal and non-steroidal molecules. The steroidal anti-androgens are best represented by cyproterone acetate. They interfere with the nuclear androgen receptor, block 5 alpha reductase but also display a progesteron-type antigonadotrophic activity. They are regarded as adequate monotherapy, but carry the stigma of cardiovascular toxicity as the other steroid drugs [35].

The second group of anti-androgens displaces T from the androgen receptor, not only in the prostate but also at the level of the hypothalamus, with a subsequent increase of LH secretion resulting in a rise in serum T.

There was concern that this rise in serum T could override the blocking effects of the pure anti-androgens, but clinical studies have demonstrated adequate responses to flutamide and casodex as monotherapy. This blocking effect in the face of a rising serum T has been demonstrated in clinical studies by giving flutamide and nilutamide in addition to monotherapy of LHRH A to prevent a possible transient clinical flare.

The toxicity of the anti-androgens concerns gastro-intestinal disturbances, hepatic toxicity and gynaecomastia in up to 10% of the treated cases for flutamide, while hemeralopia is a problem with nilutamide. Casodex, due to its pharmacokinetic properties, carries the least toxicity, but few randomised trials have been completed to draw a definitive conclusion on its clinical potential as monotherapy in prostate cancer. The most interesting aspect of these drugs is their ability to maintain potency in treated patients.

Most of the clinical interest has been centred on the addition of the pure anti-androgens to orchiectomy or monotherapy with LHRH A to provide not only cover against the physiological rise in serum T, but a permanent cover against the circulating adrenal androgens. This concept has been pursued since the original work of Huggins and surgical adrenalectomy, hypophysectomy, prednisone and steroid blockers of the adrenal androgen pathway as aminoglutethimide have all been tried with marginal success in patients with prostate cancer in relapse. The same rates of response, 5 to 10% objective and 10 to 20% subjective responses, have been recorded by the addition of the pure anti-androgens in this stage of the disease. Maximal androgen withdrawal and blocking treatment move this possible advantage upfront at the time of the initial diagnosis. A few phase II studies reporting improved responses and survival have been published, but the issue is not resolved by the review of the open or closed phase III trials comparing monotherapy to a form of this combination treatment. Recently, Crawford et al. [36] reported an increase in survival for patients treated by combination treatment as compared to those patients treated with daily injections of an LHRH A. However, all known randomised trials were presented in a recent workshop [37] and only a few trials showed increased survival, while the great majority of the trials out of 17 presented showed no difference in time to survival. The consensus was reached that all trials examined should be analysed for prognostic factors and be subjected to a meta-analysis to define a still possible but small advantage in survival. Of utmost interest is the open randomised trial organised by the National Cancer Institute where 1200 patients will be randomised between bilateral orchiectomy and bilateral orchiectomy with flutamide 3 x 250 mg/day. On the basis of the results of 5 randomised trials on prostate cancer, the EORTC took the next step and opened randomised trials reserved for patients with good and poor prognostic factors. Patients with good prognostic factors are eligible for no treatment, anti-androgens or bilateral orchiectomy. Patients with poor prognostic factors are eligible to medical or surgical castration with or without chemotherapy. Maturation of all these data will be analysed for a final position on the choice of endocrine treatment.

In conclusion, one may state that we have a series of first-line endocrine treatments available, but none of the regimens seems to produce significant improvements in patient survival. It is clear that none of these treatments will ever cure disseminated prostate cancer. It is therefore an obligation to tailor the treatment to the individual patient based on his conceptions of his quality of life compared to the anticipated side effects which do include the cost of treatment. A scheme of the different choices is presented in Table 6 as a rough guide to the selection of the first-line treatment. It is the responsibility of the urologist to integrate the patient's conception into the decision-making process after evaluation of the stage, the general condition of the patient and the prognostic factors. Even then, this obligation is carried through the follow-up where interim prognostic factors may suggest a change in surveillance frequency or therapy [38].

Second-Line Alternative Treatment

Essentially, all patients who responded to first-line hormonal treatment relapsed by progression of the primary tumour and/or its metastases to a state where the hormone unresponsive cancer cells dominate the clini-

Table 6. Treatment selection according to the conception of the patient

Patient's conception	Possible treatment choice
No surgery	LHRH A (anti-androgens) Oestrogens Anti-androgens (experimental)
No mutilation/No gynaecomastia	Subcapsular orchiectomy Pretreatment radiation LHRH A
No impotence	Pure anti-androgens Trial period of reversible LHRH A treatment
Indifferent to sexual status	Bilateral orchiectomy
Cardiovascular risk	No oestrogens
Treatment efficacy reservation	Trial treatment with LHRH A

cal picture. Simple single endocrine treatment as bilateral orchiectomy only produces a response if the first-line treatment has failed to bring the testosterone down to castrate levels [39]. No responses have been reported with the addition of LHRH A treatment.

Marginal and brief responses have been reported by the addition of oestrogens, banking on the presumed cytotoxic effects. Beneficial, especially subjective, responses have been reported by the administration of high doses of diethylstilboestrol-diphosphate [40]. Also, high doses of MPA have been shown to produce some activity in these cases and treatment superiority to prednisone was reported [41]. Reliable response rates have been reported in the order of 30% for high-dose estramustine phosphate, which provides simultaneously an oestrogenic and cytotoxic action. Side effects, especially in these debilitated patients, are common. The combination of prednisone with nor-nitrogen mustard is under investigation.

The question arises when prostate cancer becomes refractory to hormonal treatment: is it safe to stop the first-line treatment? We know that hormone unresponsiveness of the tumour in this stage is a misnomer, since the administration of exogeneous testosterone brings a host of side effects in about 80% of these patients [42].

Simple logic dictates a solution where serum T is kept at castrate levels. This is easily achieved by converting any therapy to bilateral orchiectomy.

The institution of combination treatment, usually by adding an anti-androgen to monotherapy, received praise for the early results, but came quickly down to a sobering 7% objective response and an additional 15% subjective response. Along with this concept came the use of drugs able to suppress the adrenal androgen steroidogenesis. Aminoglutethimide (AG) completely suppresses adrenal function, requiring substitution of cortisone. The amelioration is mostly subjective with a decrease of pain. Ketoconazole (K) is more selective in its interference with the adrenal steroidogenesis. A definite further suppression of serum T is noted which resulted in pain relief in a number of patients for a brief period of time. The clinical application was discontinued because of reports of adrenal insufficiency. The side effects include gastro-intestinal intolerance with nausea and vomiting [43].

A new derivative of imidazole looks more promising in the phase I/II trials with objective and subjective responses in a first series of patients [44]. This positive effect was not due to the lowering of the adrenal androgens, but to raised tissue levels of retinoic acid as an effective mechanism. Somatostatine (SMS) has shown some effect on tumour growth in the Dunning R 3327 prostate cancer model and its clinical investigation is in progress.

Extensive efforts by all clinical research groups led by the National Prostatic Cancer Project (USA) to identify effective chemotherapeutic agents failed so far to select first choices comparable to estramustine phosphate. The survival curves of all single agents in a composite graph of all curves, which we call the spaghetti curves, gives an immediate appreciation of the lack of progress in this search. Combination treatments between conventional chemotherapy, chemotherapy and endocrine therapy, do not improve this picture. The currently used drugs which demonstrated over 20% of responses are presented in Table 7.

Table 7. Single agents with reasonable response rates in men with relapsed prostate cancer

Doxorubicin	Estramustine
Epirubicin	Mitomycine C
Cyclophosphamide	Vinblastine
Cisplatin	

At this moment, it is wise to stick to single agents. Some have been reported to be effective in low repetitive doses to avoid excessive toxicity which is to be expected in these patients. A recent newcomer in this group is suramin, which has been shown to inhibit different tissue growth factors, one of which, the fibroblast growth factor (FGF), is present in prostate cancer. We obtained 35% short-term responses in a small group of heavily pretreated patients. The drug toxicity and its pharmacokinetic spectrum are under study before phase II studies can be undertaken [45]. The clinical results do not support any state of the art chemotherapy in prostate cancer, but it seems the only rational way to improve on the overall treatment of prostate cancer in relapse.

Conclusions

Progress in treatment results depends largely on the discovery of new drugs or new treatments, treatment preferences based on clearcut results of randomised clinical trials, an outstanding patient selection based on prognostic factors and the characteristics of patient and disease alike.

Controversy abounds, due to a number of factors among which the most important ones are:

1. Our failure to appreciate the biological activity of the tumour in the individual patient;
2. Our lack of consensus on aspects of staging, response, initial and intermittent prognostic factors;
3. Our problem to calculate the risk of concomitant diseases;
4. Our lack of understanding of the relativity of phase II trial results and the controversy flowing from different end results of phase III trials.

We are not quite capable of presenting spectacular results in all of these problems, but we can state with confidence that the urologists have laboured to comprehend the complexity of this heterogeneous disease. The results of several consensus meetings organised on a worldwide scale to utilise identical criteria, to collaborate on the analysis of clinical trials and to invest time in linking basic research to patient care, give reason for optimism. Progress in treatment comes in small quantum at the time and we are confident in predicting that we will settle the controversy on endocrine treatment before the next century. Our common goal is to provide years to live for our patients, which is exactly our guidance for further clinical research.

REFERENCES

1 Murphy GP, Natarajan N, Pontes JE, Schmitz RL, Schmidt JD, Mettlin C: The national survey of prostate cancer in the United States by the American College of Surgeons. J Urol 1982 (127):928-934
2 Office of Medical Applications of Research, National Institutes of Health, Bethesda: The management of clinically, localised prostate cancer. J Am Med Ass 1987 (258):2727-2730
3 Denis L: The Medical Management of Prostatic Cancer-Monograph. European School of Oncology. Heidelberg, Springer-Verlag 1988
4 Cantrell BB, Deklerk DP, Eggleston JC, Boitnott JK, Walsh PC: Pathological factors that influence prognosis in stage A prostatic cancer: The influence of extent versus grade. J Urol 1981 (125):516-520
5 Hermanek P, Sobin LH: TNM Classification of Malignant Tumours. International Union against Cancer, Geneva 1987, 4th edition
6 Gervasi LA, Mata J, Easly JD, Wilbanks JH, Seale-Hawkins C, Carlton CE Jr, Scardino PT: Prognostic significance of lymph nodal metastases in prostate cancer. J Urol 1989 (142):332-336
7 Smith PH, Bono A, Calais da Silva F, Debruyne F, Denis L, Robinson P, Sylvester R, Armitage TG, Members of the EORTC Urological Group: Some limitations of the radioisotope bone scan in patients with metastatic prostatic cancer: A sub-analysis of EORTC trial 30853. Cancer 1990 (66,5 Suppl):3-10
8 Mc Neal JE: The prostate gland: Morphology and pathobiology. In: Stamey TA (ed) Monographs in Urology: Prostate. Custom Publishing Services, Princeton 1988 pp 36-54
9 Jewett HJ, Bridge RW, Gray GF, Shelley WM: The palpable nodule of prostatic cancer. JAMA 1968 (203):403-406
10 Graversen PH, Gasser TC, Madsen PO, Corle DK: Early prostatic cancer: radical prostatectomy versus placebo. J Urol 1987 (131):364A
11 Van Aubel OGJM, Hoekstra WJ, Schroeder FH: Early orchiectomy for patients with stage D1 prostatic carcinoma. J Urol 1985 (134):292-294
12 Denis L: Current trends in prostatic cancer care. In: Furr BJA, Denis L (eds) Clinical Oncology: Prostate Cancer: International Practice and Research. Bailliäre Tindall, London 1988 2(3) pp 675-686
13 Newling D, Fossa S, Tunn U, Kurth KH, De Pauw M, Sylvester R, Members of the EORTC GU Group: Preliminary results of phase III study of mitomycin C versus estramustine in progressive metastatic prostate cancer refractory to hormonal therapy: Results of EORTC GU Group Study 30865. Eur Urol 1990 (18-suppl.1):2
14 Whitmore WW: Clinical management of prostatic cancer: An overview. Am J Clin Oncol (CCT) 1988 (11-Suppl 2):88-97
15 Gleason DF: Histologic grading and clinical staging of prostatic carcinoma. In: Tannenbaum M (ed) Urologic Pathology: The Prostate. Lea & Febiger, Philadelphia 1977 (part II) pp 171-198
16 Standaert B, Van Der Auwera JC, Chaban M, Cornet A, Eylenbosch W, Denis L: The use of transrectal echography for screening on prostate cancer: Results and evaluation. In: Murphy GP, Khoury S, Kuss R, Chatelain C, Denis L (eds) Prostate cancer Part B: Imaging techniques, radiotherapy, chemotherapy, and management issues. AR Liss, New York 1987 pp 29-36
17 Braeckman J, Denis L: The practice and pitfalls of ultrasonography in the lower urinary tract. Eur Urol 1983 (9):193-201
18 Lee F, Torp-Pedersen ST, Siders DB, Kumasaka GH, McHugh TA: The use of transrectal ultrasound in the study of normal and abnormal anatomy of the prostate gland. In: Labrie F, Lee F, Dupont A (eds) Diagnosis and Choice of Therapy: Early Stage Prostate Cancer. Elsevier Sci Publ, Amsterdam 1989 pp 23-36
19 Cooper EH, Armitage TH, Robinson MRG, Newling DWW, Richards BR, Smith PH, Denis L, Sylvester R: Prostatic specific antigen and the prediction of prognosis in metastatic prostatic cancer. Cancer 1989 (66,5-Suppl):19-22
20 Schröder FH, Cooper EH, Debruyne FMJ et al: TNM classification of genitourinary tumours 1987. Position of EORTC Genitourinary Group. Br J Urol 1988 (62):502-510
21 Jones WG: Can the primary tumour be used as the sole parameter for response in phase II chemotherapy studies in metastatic prostate cancer? An EORTC Genito-Urinary Group Report. World J Urol 1986 (4):176-181
22 Denis L, Mettlin C: Conclusions. Proceedings workshop on combined castration and androgen blockade therapy in prostate cancer: Results and future directions. Cancer 1990 (66,5-suppl):80-83
23 Mettlin C, Denis L: Introduction. Proceedings workshop on combined castration and androgen blockade therapy in prostate cancer: Results and future directions. Cancer 1990 (66,5-suppl):2
24 Kirk D: Trial and tribulations in prostate cancer. Br J Urol 1987 (59):375-379
25 Altwein J: Estrogen in the treatment of prostate cancer. In: Pavone Macaluso M, Smith PH (eds) Cancer of the Prostate and Kidney. Plenum Press, New York 1983 pp 317-328
26 Denis L: Current trends in prostatic care. In: Furr BJA, Denis L (eds) Clinical Oncology: Prostate Cancer: International Practice and Research. Balliäre Tindall, London 1988 (2,3) pp 675-686
27 Aro J, Haapiainen R, Sane T, Rannikko S, Pelkonen R, Alfthan O: Effects of orchiectomy and polyestradiol phosphate therapy on serum lipoprotein lipids and glucose tolerance in prostatic cancer patients. Eur Urol 1989 (636):1-11
28 Smith PH, Suciu S, Robinson MRG, Richards B, Bastable JRG, Glashan RW, Bouffioux C, Lardennois B, Williams RE, De Pauw M, Sylvester R: A comparison of the effect of diethylstilbestrol and low dose estramustine phosphate in the treatment of advanced prostatic cancer: A phase II trial of the EORTC Urological Group. J Urol 1986 (136):619-623
29 Furr BJA, Milsted RAV: LHRH analogues in cancer treatment. In: Stoll BA (ed) Endocrine Management of Cancer 2: Contemporary Therapy. Karger, Basel 1988 pp 16-29

30 Denis L: Analogues de la LHRH. In: Khoury S, Chatelain C (eds) Urologie: Cancer de la Prostate. FIIS, Paris 1988 pp 351-359
31 Newling DWW: The value of reversible androgen suppression as a diagnostic test. In: Murphy GP, Khoury S, Küss R, Chatelain C, Denis L (eds) Prostate Cancer Part A: Research, Endocrine Treatment and Histopathology. AR Liss, New York 1987 pp 261-265
32 Namer M: Rationale for medical castration. In: Furr BJA, Denis L (eds) Clinical Oncology: Prostate Cancer: International Practice and Research. Bailliäre Tindall, London 1988 pp 535-546
33 Blackard CE: The Veterans Administration Cooperative Urological Research Group studies of carcinoma of the prostate: A review. Cancer Chemother Reports1975 (59):225-227
34 Haapiainen R, Rannikko S, Alfthan O: Comparison of primary orchiectomy with oestrogen therapy in advanced prostatic cancer: A 2 year follow-up report of a national, prospective prostatic cancer study. Brit J Urol 1986 (58):528-533
35 Jacobi H, Neumann F: The Case for Cyproterone Acetate. Clinical Oncology: Prostate Cancer: International Practice and Research. Bailliäre Tindall, London 1988 2(3) pp 571-580
36 Crawford DE, Eisenberger MA, Mcleod D, Spaulding JT, Benson R, Dorr FA, Blumenstein BA, Davis MA, Goodman PJ: A controlled trial of leuprolide with and without flutamide in prostatic carcinoma. N Engl J Med 1989 (321):419-424
37 Denis L, Murphy G, Dalesio O: Workshop on a meta-analysis of trials involving combination treatment in prostatic cancer. Paris 1990
38 Suciu S, Sylvester RJ, Yamanaka H: Time-dependent prognostic factors in advanced prostatic cancer. In: Newling DWW, Jones WG (eds) Prostate Cancer and Testicular Cancer. Wiley-Liss, New York 1990 pp 203-215
39 Keuppens F, Fossa S, Nowé P, Denis L: Secondary orchiectomy in patients with prostatic cancer in relapse. In: Denis L, Murphy GP, Prout GR, Schröder FH (eds) Controlled Clinical Trials in Urologic Oncology. Raven Press, New York 1984 pp 207-209
40 Denis L, Murphy G, Droz P: Personal communication
41 Fossa SD, Ogreid P, Karlsen S, Havelan H, Jensen J, Trovag A: High dose medroxyprogesterone acetate (MPA) versus prednisolone (P) in hormone-resistant prostate cancer. In: Bracci U, Di Silverio F (eds) Advances in Urological Oncology and Endocrinology. Acta Medica, Rome 1984 pp 433-437
42 Denis L, Mahler C: LHRH agonist combination treatment. In: Motta M, Serio M (eds) Hormonal Therapy of Prostatic Diseases: Basic and Clinical Aspects. Medicom, Amsterdam 1987 pp 85-92
43 Mahler C: Ketoconazole. In: Khoury S, Chatelain C (eds) Urologie: Cancer de la Prostate. FIIS, Paris 1988 pp 365-368
44 Denis L, Mahler C, Ongena P, Janssen P, De Coster R, Bruynseels J: A phase I/II study with R75251, a novel imidazole derivative in M1 prostate cancer patients in relapse. Abstract IXth Congress of the European Association of Urology, Amsterdam, 1990
45 Van Oosterom AT, De Smedt EA, Denis LJ, de Bruijn EA, Mahler C: Suramine for prostatic cancer: A phase I/II study in advanced extensively pretreated disease. EJC 1990 (26,4):422

FSC
www.fsc.org
MIX
Papier aus verantwortungsvollen Quellen
Paper from responsible sources
FSC® C105338

If you have any concerns about our products,
you can contact us on
ProductSafety@springernature.com

In case Publisher is established outside the EU,
the EU authorized representative is:
Springer Nature Customer Service Center GmbH
Europaplatz 3, 69115 Heidelberg, Germany

Printed by Libri Plureos GmbH
in Hamburg, Germany